BOUNCING BACK FROM MULTIPLE SCLEROSIS

G. PATRICK MCINTIRE

BOUNCING BACK FROM MULTIPLE SCLEROSIS

ISBN: 1-4196-9789-7
Library of Congress Control Number: 20008904375
BookSurge Publishing
G. Patrick McIntire
www.bouncingbackfromms.com
425-831-5818
E mail: bounceback@centurytel.net

Cover Design: Kim Starr
Beachball at Koloa Point – Oil painting on canvas by Kim Starr
www.kimstarrgallery.com

This book is intended to serve only as a resource. I cannot assume medical or legal responsibility of having the contents of this book considered as a prescription for anyone. Treatment of health disorders needs to be supervised by your physician or licensed health care professional.

CONTENTS PAGE

ACKNOWLEDGMENT AND DEDICATION

This book is dedicated to my wonderful Mother and Father. All their nurturing and love has made my healing possible. "Long on enthusiasm" my Father would say. This had to come from somewhere.

"I give my mind and body the tools, the time and the desire to heal."
                                                                    Author

Introduction

BOUNCING BACK FROM MULTIPLE SCLEROSIS
By G. Patrick McIntire

No hypodermic needles please, before you read this book. *Bouncing Back from Multiple Sclerosis* **is** based on fourteen years of diaries I kept since being diagnosed with MS in October of 1990. I developed a daily program for living with MS without the use of injectable drugs. Approximately 400,000 Americans acknowledge having MS. Every week about 200 people are diagnosed. MS may affect 2.5 million individuals worldwide.

Through this book I am offering you a gift of fourteen years of personal experience with MS. It is my hope that the information compiled in this diary will inspire you to seek and find alternative methods for living a quality life with Multiple Sclerosis. I share in this book information on vitamins, exercises, meditation, and a modified lifestyle routine. The title of this book is a perfect fit for this disease. Bouncing back is what we all strive for. In 1990 there were no injectable disease modifying drugs for Multiple Sclerosis approved by the Food and Drug Administration. By sheer timing I was cast into the world of MS like many others without a clue on how to begin dealing with this unpredictable disease. There was no Copaxone, Rebif, Betaseron or Avonex available to prescribe. In 1990, I was so sick and scared I would have signed up for one of the injectable disease modifying drugs if my Medical Doctor had suggested I do so. I would have given myself the injections or paid a weekly visit to the Doctor for the Avonex injection. I would have somehow come up with the $1000 per month for the injectable drugs.

Readers of this book today have the choices I did not have. The disease modifying drugs are now available. All the advertising by the drug manufacturers are set in place to attract the MS patient to their drug. ***Bouncing Back from Multiple Sclerosis*** is a must read before jumping into making "your choice" for a disease modifying drug. There are many of us living with MS that do not use disease modifying drugs and never have. ***Bouncing Back from Multiple Sclerosis*** is my story.

As my father and mother would say, "Do your homework."

Forward

It's not often that a complete stranger walks up to you and offers a gift but that is exactly what G. Patrick McIntire is doing for you with "Bouncing Back." He is offering the gift of his experience with multiple sclerosis that can change your life. He reveals how the devastating news of his condition left him feeling stunned with little comfort or understanding as to how his life would be affected.

Seventeen years ago Patrick was diagnosed with MS. This was a time when little was known about the disease, and less about treatment or cure. In the following chapters Patrick reveals how he came to grips with the fear of never being the same again.

So began the search for information that would enable him to overcome, or at least learn to live a productive life with MS. There are no words to express the fear, loneliness and abandonment one feels after being diagnosed with a debilitating disease, nor are these words necessary, because it is such a personal experience, *your* experience.

Embrace Patrick's gift, let each chapter unfold and reveal to you the benefit of his experience. Today Patrick is a very productive, active and loving survivor who has met the horror of the diagnosis of MS. Today he is offering you options that are alternative to drug therapies not available seventeen years ago. He is not saying drugs do not work; it is more like having an alternative natural method, with no side effects and certainly not the cost.

Know that as long as there are friends out there like Patrick, you are never alone. Let him guide you through the labyrinth of the unknown, and into the light of understanding and love. It may be true, you will never be the same, but with Patrick's help, you can be better.

L.W. Shortridge, PhD

PREFACE   I could be President…that will have to wait.

Never in my wildest dreams would I have thought I would have Multiple Sclerosis. I did not even know what it was until I was faced with the diagnosis. Yes, I had only heard the words with no meaning.

This situation changed abruptly in 1990. From then on I was living with the diagnosis of Multiple Sclerosis. MS was never far from my psyche or physical body since. Life had changed for me. I began living with symptoms that drained the fun right out of my life. I was not aware these symptoms ever existed. Who made these up? I don't like this. I was until then, strong, Aries, left handed and smart. I could have been president.

Instead I was struggling with a myriad of symptoms that would not leave my body and mind alone. Remember I reminded myself, I was left handed, and I could be president. Not now maybe but later I reassured myself.

So I continued to whirl with vertigo, loss of bowel control, scared to go to bed for fear I would wake up with strobes instead of sight like I did last month.

It appeared this host body and mind is going to be learning some new lessons and from the way I was feeling I needed to hold on to as much reality as I could. The symptoms I was experiencing at that time did not even seem like me. Well, I was still me but things were changing.

A Note from the Author

Many times I wish I wasn't the one writing in a journal all these years. Times in the early years of life with MS were full of symptoms, trauma, anguish, fear, and the unknown future. Yet these journals continue to be my road map for the past, present and future.

I live fully with Multiple Sclerosis. I have turned these writings into chapters containing my health regimen, synapse of diaries, foods I consume, exercises I rely on and my basic life tools I use for living with MS.

As you read this book expect to read more books. Your literary journey about MS has probably just begun. I have penned part of my journey in this book. You will feel empowerment when you begin forming your own game plan and writing your plan down. Whoever you are, take control. NOW.

To journey into the writings of a book is fulfillment. A very welcome feeling when trying to ignore Multiple Sclerosis symptoms. If you are in the throes of MS and find comfort in this book, I will be fulfilled.

Author

Cellular Change

After reading *Ann Boroch's* book, *"Healing Multiple Sclerosis,"* published in 2007, I was quite taken back by her writing on MS. Not only is her book a must read for anyone associated with Multiple Sclerosis, the book also makes me revisit my own healing journey. *Ann Boroch* points out the importance of every cell having a memory on page 84 and on to the effects of joy and laughter on page 160.

The first time I heard of cells each having memory was in *Dr. Chopra's* book, "Quantum Healing." A particular chapter titled, "Ghosts of memory." This means the trillions of cells that each of us are composed of respond to change. Both positive and negative. How? Power of positive thinking perhaps? The euphemism I created to comfort and keep my mind positive.

"I give my mind and body the tools, the time and the desire to heal." I said these words thousands and thousands of times for many of my healing years. I was hurting, grasping, praying, all these feelings were upon me. Many times the two steps forward in healing and one step back was an hourly experience. Yet after a year or so I was having more success finding a half hour here and an hour there with a relief of symptoms. This relief. What is it? Cellular change?

After reading *Dr. Deepak Chopra* and many others and now *Ann Boroch*, I believe this is what happened to me. A cellular change. A healing cell to cell. I can do it. So can you.

Shock and Relief
Diagnosis

The awe of a diagnosis of Multiple Sclerosis comes to each of us at a time when we are physically and mentally in a very vulnerable state. I will never forget this event in my own life. The violent attack that woke me up and immediately sent me to the doctor didn't yet have a name. Doctors needed to do more tests to uncover the mystery. I am sure each doctor may have held back a guess or two. But doctors would rather not guess and be wrong. I agree. In other words they often know enough to recognize how little they really do know.

I was having significant vertigo and balance problems. So the tests continued. My primary care physician thought from the beginning I may be dealing with an inner ear infection. Thus the vertigo and balance problems. Yet what I was going through every minute of every day didn't seem like something as simple as an ear infection. I had never had an ear infection but doesn't something with the word "infection" mean you take antibiotics and it goes away?

This showed me how uninformed I was about what was happening to me. My doctor sent me home and said it should clear up in a few days or weeks at most. But this malady did not clear up. It remained scary. I remember moving a load of top soil in the neighbor's back yard over the fence to our yard. Wheel barrow after wheel barrow. Shovel after shovel. Hoping the never ending symptoms would just go away. Yet the symptoms stayed with me no matter how hard I worked and no matter how much water I drank. I could not work the symptoms off. I remained very concerned. Freaked out actually.

Of course words like brain tumor came to mind. This was probably due to watching too much television. I had a feeling this was bigger than an inner ear infection. So I decided to go see a naturopathic physician. The physician had a look and decided to treat my symptoms with a homeopathic treatment. Which means "like treating like." This made the symptoms even worse. Of course this is what is supposed to happen except the patient is supposed to improve after the treatment.

Not me. A week went by and I decided to see another medical doctor. After a physical which included reflex response, the doctor said he did not have any definitive diagnosis but obviously something is really bothering me. "Would you like to see a Neurologist?" he asked. "Yes!" I answered. I made an appointment.

By then I was really reacting badly and felt terrible as well. I arrived at the neurologist's office. The neurologist gave me an exam. After completion he said he did not have a definitive diagnosis but obviously something was really bothering me. He suggested scheduling a magnetic resonating image scan (MRI) done on my brain. My answer was a resounding yes. The neurologist asked when and I said right now.

I don't know about you but volunteering for anything in a doctor's office is not something I would normally do. This just shows you how bad I felt. I needed to find out what was wrong with me. Then at least I could absorb the news, good or bad, and go from there.

As I reflect back on this decision I remember the first bit of hope, mixed with fear. Relief came from the realization that the last month, tormenting as it was, served as a catalyst to discover a true diagnosis, good, bad or ugly. I felt like I was dying.

So I needed an answer at least. I knew nothing can feel like this and have a good outcome. But I had to put a name to the malady and I had to know as soon as possible. The MRI scan was set up for the same evening. I made arrangements to stay in a hotel once I found out I would be given a sedative before beginning the test. The procedure was painless but I had to lie perfectly still for the hour it took to image my brain with the scanner. The test itself went fine.

I anxiously waited for the neurologist to call. When he did he told me I did not have a brain tumor but they knew what was wrong with me and I should come into review the diagnosis. I entered the neurologist office once again. During the consultation he told me "You have Multiple Sclerosis." I really felt like whatever I was dealing with was critical and closing in on me very quickly. But not knowing the effects of Multiple Sclerosis, all I could do is ask "What is Multiple Sclerosis?" The doctor proceeded to explain the disease. Then I asked him what I could do.

First, stay out of the heat because this makes symptoms more pronounced, there is no cure and there is no treatment. Remember, this was 1990 and conventional allopathic medicine had yet to offer drugs to treat MS except certain and specific symptoms. Of which were not a long term protocol for MS patients.

He said I could possibly live a natural life and never have another episode or I could experience episodes in the future. No one knows. There was little comfort in his prognosis. One additional tidbit of information the doctor left me with. **It rarely kills anybody.**

This whole experience left me with more questions than answers. I called my medical doctor immediately to tell him the news! Knowing that he would be one to perhaps explain some options for me if anyone could. This consultation became a benchmark in my healing.

My doctor laid out options where the neurologist had none and said Western medicine had nothing for me and suggested I research Eastern medicine and philosophy. Now I felt like I was getting somewhere. Finding options was all I was asking for by this time. I understood there was no cure and I accepted the danger of the disease. But there had to be options out there to improve my condition.

This is exactly how I looked at what *Dr. Douwe Rienstra* was telling me. There is hope. Always. No matter how screwed up I was or will be I can live and re-achieve a quality of life both physically and mentally. I learned to mentally and physically live with Multiple Sclerosis. Minute by minute, day by day.

What would I do now if I was just diagnosed with MS

T The question: What would I do now if I was just diagnosed with MS? Twelve painless and inexpensive steps. These early steps made a huge difference in my healing.

1. Begin a journal now.

The mechanics of writing in your journal has *you* becoming involved in the process of living with MS. You are now better able to assist in present and future decisions you will have to make. As you live your life with MS you can refer to your journal as a research tool.

When was the last time I consumed dairy? When did I add fish oil to my supplement regimen? What dosage? What about Vitamin D? What day did I begin an exercise program?

These answers and others from now on can be found in your journal. To have this record whether a day or week or a year old is empowerment.

This information is your information. You can choose to share this information in an informative way with your family or doctor. It is your choice. You are contributing to your health from now on.

2. Find an MD that is confident and familiar with alternative solutions to specific situations when appropriate. I was fortunate to have *Dr. Douwe Rienstra* in my town when I was first diagnosed. *Dr. Rienstra* is an M.D. with additional specialized training in Ayurvedic Medical sciences. *Dr. Rienstra* and doctors with similar interests in healing simply have extra tools in their healing tool box. Remember they are supposed to be working for and with you in your quest to heal and live with Multiple Sclerosis. The steps are painless. Yet the impact for a person newly diagnosed can be significant. I can hear people saying to themselves "how do I begin?" You must transform the paradigm from "what am I to do" to "what am I doing".

3. Learn to breathe properly. A simple five minute exercise known as *pranayama* is shown in *"Perfect Health"* by *Dr. Deepak Chopra*. Learning this simple technique can enhance and hasten your healing. Remember you do not have to be in a doctor's office to practice this healing technique. When you are stressed, you become fatigued. This is a good time to balance your breathing for relief. Pranayama will become second nature to you. This technique is *free* for you to use anytime of the day or night.

4. My medical doctor taught me *Transcendental Meditation*. I paid a fee for the classes. My doctor also provided free of charge a continued opportunity to check my progress in meditation technique. *Dr. Chopra's* books and *Dr. Weil's* books and others illustrate meditation techniques. Learn meditation as soon as possible.

5. Stop using dairy of any kind immediately. I was six months past the formal diagnosis of MS when I got a hold of *John Pageler's* book *"New Hope Real Help for People with MS"*. John's book is now out of print. An emphatic statement leaped off the pages at me. *Stop using*

dairy! I was having real intestinal (bowel) issues at this time, with many incidences of lack of control, to many humiliating near misses and lots of discomfort and bowel looseness. John's book suggested that dairy could be associated with causing these bowel symptoms. By eliminating dairy (and I did not cheat) most of us drop a significant amount of "saturated fat" immediately out of our daily diet. Read books about your heart health and dropping saturated fat out of the diet is the right way to go whether you make the change for your heart or for living with MS. This is the first step in modifying your diet.

6. Stop consuming foods containing sugar immediately. Please question every item that is headed to your mouth for potential fuel. Your digestion system does not need extra challenges at this juncture. We are working on healing and balancing. Now is the time to practice your willpower. The more you slip, the longer it will take to get on top of your life with MS.

7. Practice a self sesame oil massage known as *abhyanga* in Ayurvedic medicine. *Dr. Chopra* in his book *"Perfect Health"* illustrates this technique. I gave myself a daily sesame oil massage for several years. I wish everyone that reads this book will follow Dr Chopra's writings and learn sesame oil massage immediately! To this day, knowing what I have physically gone through I can say without question sesame oil massage on countless occasions was the only thing I had to look forward to from one day to the next. Did it relieve symptoms? You Bet! Did the massage help my breathing? You bet! Did sesame oil massage help my circulation? You bet. Did it feel good? You bet! Do I feel sesame oil massage is a must? Yes I do! Begin today!

8. Use a Candida cleanse immediately. A book I read early on while in the throes of symptoms titled *"The Yeast Connection"* by *Dr. William Crook MD* points out the potential overgrowth of Candida albicans in all Multiple Sclerosis patients. Sugar feeds this unwelcome imbalance. There are inexpensive supplements at health food stores to support the elimination of Candida in your system. Lethargy and foggy thought

senses are a couple of the symptoms that can point to an overgrowth of Candida in the system.

9. Pay attention to your protein intake and make sure this is kept at feel good levels. During the early years of MS I found consuming a protein source every couple of hours worked for me. I have always been very thin in stature. An example snack would be a boiled egg with a dash of salt and a little mustard.

10. Read "*Creating Health*", "*Quantum Healing*" and "*Perfect Health*" by *Dr. Deepak Chopra*. Enjoy reading these books one day at a time. Take notes in your journal as you follow *Dr. Chopra's* words. This is a part of taking control of your day to day routine. *Dr. Chopra* is an MD and Endocrinologist and also Ayurvedic (Eastern medicine) trained physician. These books are important tools in many ways. I found great strength in these words. Each page adds to *Dr. Chopra's* convincing theory on mind body capabilities. Once you have read "*Creating Health*" and "*Quantum Healing*" you will want to add "*Perfect Health*" by *Dr. Chopra* to your book of tools. This book will explain techniques to enhance your opportunities to change and heal. Actually, read everything you can get your hands on about MS. In my own healing I put *Dr. Chopra's* books in this top category for many reasons. You will be well served when you open any of these books. Start taking notes, and use them as your reference library, the sooner the better. I realize at this particular time your symptoms may be overwhelming. This is why *Dr. Chopra's* books are so important to you and to me. These books lay out a philosophy of health that has been taught for thousands of years. And is finally catching on in the west. For people like us there are few if any alternatives at the pharmacy or doctors office. What you can expect from *Dr. Chopra's* books are techniques to deal with many of the symptoms of MS and other imbalances. From there you can formulate your techniques to hasten your healing.

11. Read "*Healing Multiple Sclerosis*" by *Ann Boroch* and "*The Multiple Sclerosis Diet Book*" by *Dr. Roy Swank*, a Neurologist. Both excellent books with many insights to diet and living with MS. *Ann Boroch* being diagnosed with MS herself is a great inspiration to all of us. *Dr.Swank* points out by following the precepts developed over the years, a great majority of patients can expect to remain free of disability for over thirty-five years if his methods are initiated before the disability has developed. Reading the first 108 pages will convince you to pay attention to what *Dr. Swank* has to offer people with a diagnosis of MS. Remember, *Dr. Swank* maintains his beliefs and so do I. *Dr. Swank* published his first paper "*Multiple Sclerosis: A correlation*" in conventional medical literature in 1950 and remained active as a neurologist for many years after this literature was published. He describes MS in language that can be understood. And in a straightforward way that gave me hope. *Dr. Swank's* main belief is a low fat diet is absolutely critical in dealing with MS. I can remember how much support his positivity and certainty gave me. Now when I look at the recipes that follow the first 108 pages of *Dr. Swank's* book I realized by purchasing the same basic foods over and over again I could prepare and cook foods simpler than *Dr. Swank*. By the way, *Dr. Swank* allows skim milk in his diet for MS. I do not like skim milk so it is easier for me to just say *No Dairy*. The general premise of *Dr. Swank's* Diet Book for MS is a simple approach to a complex disease. A diet change can prove to be difficult in that it may eliminate some of your favorite foods. This is not consistent mainstream medical thinking of drug therapy which often seems to regard diseases as drug deficiencies. Drugs tend to alleviate the symptoms, not cure the disease. Doctors may suggest that a good balanced diet is important but pretty much all the hope they offer is a hope of reducing incidence of exacerbation by about a third by choosing one of the four available FDA approved drugs.

12. Read about *Sunrider* herbs (www.sunrider.com). This is a multi level marketing company. I took the combination of herbs called the "quinary" for four years. Did they make a difference? Yes, I believe

so. I also took three other herb combinations by *Sunrider* called Top, Joi and Ese.

Chapter

3

Recap Game Plan Daily

The books and papers I studied and all the trial and error comprise these steps.

1. Begin a journal now. Date the first page. Write down your first thought. You have just begun the first step of healing and control of MS.
2. Find a doctor that will work with you in your healing.
3. Learn to breathe properly. Pranayama.
4. Learn to meditate.
5. Stop using dairy of any kind!
6. Stop consuming foods that contain sugar! Read package labels!
7. Practice sesame oil massage (Abhyanga)
   www.ayurbalance.com/explore
8. Use a Candida cleanse herb product from your health food store. Your doctor can recommend a product.
9. Eat adequate protein. Write this in your journal. Record in your journal how this meal makes you feel. This is what your journal is all about. Keeping track and improving your outcome.
10. Read *"Creating Health"* and *"Quantum Healing"* and *"Perfect Health"* by *Dr. Chopra.* www.chopra.com
11. Read *"Healing Multiple Sclerosis"* by *Ann Boroch.* www.annboroch.com and *"The Multiple Sclerosis Diet Book"* by *Dr. Roy Swank.* www.swankmsdiet.com

12. Read about *Sunrider Herbs*. www.sunrider.com A multi level marketing company. Do your homework and see if they are right for you.

Symptoms I have Experienced and Action I take for Management

- **Vertigo**

Action I take: If at all possible I just lie down, meditate, and balance breathing and rest.

My experience with vertigo lasted continuously for the first three years after diagnosis. I woke up in the morning and within ten to fifteen minutes vertigo would begin and would stay with me every day. In an attempt to regain my balance as I walked, I used a technique of touching my nose. I was checking to see if there was any change or how bad the symptom was every day. Nothing scientific here just a way to check the change in a symptom. I spent seven months in a warm, dry climate and noticed quite a drop in vertigo. I cannot say symptoms were gone I just don't remember the symptom being so prevalent in that environment. Any of us that have dealt with vertigo day in and day out do our best to live with it and mask the symptom. At times, to mask this symptom is very difficult. The afternoons are the most challenging. Sitting down did not seem to help me. I needed to lie down. Meditation does help but it is even better to lie down and close your eyes. I could usually reduce the symptom by doing this. Living in Hawaii for five years showed a marked improvement in my living with vertigo as well. It seems as if a combination of warm weather and sunlight makes a difference. Vertigo is one of the symptoms that can become omnipresent in a hurry for me. Most of the time a way for me to abate this long lasting symptom is to simply lie down and close my eyes.

- **Stress**

Action I take: Balance breathing, meditation, prayer, sesame oil massage, drink water.

From my own experiences stress is on the top of the list in bringing about MS symptoms. Early on I did not have my tool box full of the tools I mention above. Once I learned these techniques my stress level was manageable. I practice balance breathing and meditation every day.

- **Balance**

Action I take: Rest, meditation, balanced breathing, and practice.

I do not remember having any problem with balance prior to being diagnosed with MS. I rode a bicycle with no hands, I climbed trees, threw an accurate baseball pitch, ice skated and helped roof houses. Balance was something I never questioned. After my incident with a Multiple Sclerosis exacerbation this all changed. My balance became something I could not count on or take for granted anymore. Attempting to use a ladder took on a whole new meaning. I had to be very careful. I could get on a ladder. I could fake the ease of the act. But I did not trust myself anymore. I had to pay 100% attention when using a ladder again. I have never broken a bone in my life. To have a problem with balance was a new experience for me. My neurologist could see from tests I did not have very good timing but balance was never an issue until September of 1990. Balance is something I worked at improving. I was sure I could. Whether it was skill building exercises or just learning to challenge myself again on ice skates or dancing, I could improve. Balance is something I automatically correct now. I have ridden a bicycle in the last eighteen months. I am confident I can ride a bicycle now. But I would choose an area with little or no traffic. As I did on Kauai. My last bicycle adventure was riding around two square blocks a few times a week. Bravo, I am getting better!!

- **Gait**

Action I take: Stop walking and sit down. I do not have to lie down. Sitting down, resting, meditation, balance breathing, and eating works just fine.

After a half hour of sitting and resting the problem of wide gait has been lessened.

- **Bowel incontinence**

Action I take: Quit all dairy immediately. Balance breathing and practice meditation twice a day. Sesame oil massage before bathing. Practice, practice, practice.

Starting on September 3, 1990, the introduction to bowel problems began for me. I could not trust my bowels from that day on until I quit using dairy.

My brain seemed to be crossing the signals at any time without much, if any, notice. I would think I needed to use the bathroom only to be tricked again and not have to go because I just went ten minutes before.

At the same time there seemed to be immediacy to the signal. I had no choice. The symptoms or signal could have been false but I had better follow through and get close to a bathroom as soon as possible.

This situation in the first six months to a year really did not change. I felt more comfortable after the first year because of all the times I had to rehearse just in case. Whether I used the bathroom or not I had better be prepared and be at the bathroom door.

The symptom did not mimic diarrhea, like having the flu. More of a "flushing everything in my bowels", rather indiscriminate movement. My bowels were not holding back or constipated. The opposite was the norm. I quickly learned that "stress" was a trigger and made my bowels empty almost immediately.

- **Fatigue**

Action I take: Rest, meditation, balance breathing, eat protein.

To this day fatigue is a symptom I can count on daily. However, over the last fourteen years fatigue has taught me a lot about my rhythm of living. *Dr. Chopra* writes of Ayurvedic medicine and our internal clocks and rhythm. Again, I defer this to *"Perfect Health"* by *Dr. Chopra* in my situation.

When I pay attention to my rhythm throughout the day, I can do an adequate job controlling more symptoms that may appear. This was self limiting at times and was difficult to accept early on in my acceptance of MS. Especially since being a type "A" personality literally flings me into "yes I can" situations. Only to regret those three words a few minutes later.

I know I am not alone in this "jumping in" situation with other people with MS. We all do it. But through the years I have slowly learned the "jump" may have consequences. I am getting better at "just say no." Often the norm for MS is that fatigue will show up with a vengeance around 3:00 p.m. This is a great time to sit down and meditate. Do I? Well, in great MS fashion, I try to. But I am getting better at this routine again. Early on in my healing I would not miss the opportunity to meditate. But I have been too "busy" to make it a personal rule. But I am doing better. It seems that 4:00 pm is working well for a twenty minute meditation. I do well by getting up at the same time every day and going to bed every evening at the same time. If I do not, I am tempting the arrival of uncomfortable symptoms. Therefore, I try not to break my routine.

I am up by 7:30 am and in bed by 10:00 pm nearly every night. This may seem boring but I have found over the last fourteen years there is much more to life when you live on a schedule.

- **Sleeplessness**

Action I take: Balance breathing, meditation, one Tbls. Cod liver oil at lunch. Aspirin if needed, Nighty Night tea, chamomile tea, Calms Forte homeopathic.

I took an Ativan prescription anxiety and sleeping pill for the first three years after diagnosis. This symptom is directly related to my introduction to Multiple Sclerosis. I do not remember sleepless nights before MS; maybe a worried night growing up but sleeplessness was not an issue. Ativan worked like a charm.

Eleven years later with no drugs I do have some uneven nights. I say uneven because I will sleep an hour and a half then wake up. But most nights I sleep just fine. Back to the routine of waking at the same time and going to bed at the same time. I read for fifteen to thirty minutes in bed. This is usually about all I need. Bedtime teas like Nighty Night and Chamomile are a regular evening drink for me.

- **Depression**

Action I take: Balance breathing, meditation, exercise, positive books, protein. This symptom lands most often in the "unexpected" category. Growing up I had absolutely no idea what depression was. I was raised with an abundance of tools coming from a functional family and living in a healthy environment. Tools to avoid depression.

Then MS showed up. So many symptoms were coming at me every hour in the early years of MS. I really did not have the time to try to recognize if I was fighting depression or not. It would explain some of the questionable mental feelings, like, "why me?" "Will my spouse accept me if I were to become disabled, or will I be left alone to reinvent my life?

These fears were depressing. I did not want to think like that but we all have these questions looming if we have Multiple Sclerosis. What I do recognize is depression sneaks up on me. This is not a normal daily feeling for me. (Wow, I am so fortunate it is not daily.) When I say "sneaks up", I mean I will be coping with negative thinking that may wake me up in the middle of the night.

Yes, financial stress will do it every time and I will have to turn the light on and read something positive from a book at my bedside. Give myself the mental tools to get passed the negative thinking. This usually just takes time. After all, I know plenty of people who deal with much more stress than I on a daily basis. I admire their mental constitution, especially when I start feeling depressed myself.

How do they deal with their hourly situation with all the hardships they go through just to put their pants and shirt on every morning? Again, I am not one to be depressed. Thank you Mom and Dad for a loving childhood.

When the depressing thoughts show up they go away in a day or two. I do not take drugs for depression. I just wait the negative thoughts out. The book I keep in my bedroom and close at hand is *"The Power of Positive Thinking"* by *Norman Vincent Peale.* It has brought me comfort many times. Of course there is a library full of help in most every town. The internet is also available to many people as a research tool.

- **Memory and cognitive issues**

Action I take: Fish oil, meditate, rest, daily vitamins and herbs

In the morning I have no problem recounting information. My situation in the afternoon and evening is a whole different matter. The feeling of a scattered mind due to fatigue is a major factor and MS is to blame. My age is part of the equation but MS is a larger culprit. Before MS I never felt confused or had to search for words. Now I can expect this every afternoon. It is best if I just stop trying to make any decision that requires more than a yes or no answer. Even better to meditate or just lie down and take a nap.

It is amazing how meditation and a nap can help recharge oneself much like a battery. By the end of the day I really do need to hook up the mental and physical battery charger and leave it on overnight.

To look at the last fourteen years for any change in my memory, I do see change. The fatigue in memory is there every afternoon. Early on I would have the fatigue but not be so mentally compromised. I did not feel I was losing any ground morning to night. But I do now. Fortunately, I have been taking fish oil, ginkgo biloba, ashwaganda, seriphos, and multi vitamins to assist in my mental recovery through the years. I may have had a much more difficult problem if I had not been using these products. I base this on the fact I am fifty four years of age with MS and only feel mentally compromised in the afternoon and evenings. Mornings I am still ready to run this country as I see it.

- **Slurred Speech**

Action I take: Rest, meditation, balance breathing and other stress control exercises. I remember two episodes of slurred speech. The first episode occurred when I was sitting at my desk at work and quite suddenly I noticed my speech was not right. I tried to correct this, but the condition was not correctable. Every word was slurred. This lasted about a week. I remember trying to hide this from customers. This was my first experience. I had no idea what was going on. Then the slurred speech passed. Several years later and in the throes of MS symptoms I remember a couple of days that my speech was drawn. Again this went away. I have no extra tools in my toolbox for slurred speech, as of this writing, but it does seem to pass.

- **Skin tingling, tightening sensations**

Action I take: Rest, stress control, meditation, and oil massage. Sensory symptoms that include numbness and tingling have a tendency to come and go intermittently in MS. The most memorable skin sensations for me have been a tugging on the front part of my scalp like I had a hold of my hair in the front and tugging on it in a pulsating manner. Again, this symptom went away after a couple of days. This sensation has happened a half dozen times over the last fourteen years.

- **Numbness**

Action I take: Sesame oil massage, meditation, balance breathing, time heals. With numbness the incidents have been temporary and not permanent for me. I believe I have been able to avoid bigger problems with numbness because of my oil massages and meditation.

- **Eyesight weakening**

Action I take? Meditation, rest, herbs, antioxidants.

Being diagnosed with MS at forty years of age and now writing this book at fifty-four years of age, I can see plenty of differences in my eyesight. Although I have worn glasses for nearsightedness since the seventh grade, between then and now I do not remember my vision worsening. Obviously my vision has changed subtly with age, I have been told the lenses in my eyes are hardening. So I am fighting the "bifocal reality tour". I am in the denial stage and taking my glasses off to read. Then I put the glasses down and walk away. Sound familiar? Then I have to look for the glasses. Driving at night is something I avoid. The oncoming headlights are too bright. Add heavy traffic and a bit of compromised weather and I want to stay home. There is a book available which may be of some help called *"Improve Your Vision"* by *Dr. Steven M. Beresford, Dr David W. Muris, Dr. Merril J Allen and Dr. Francis A. Young.*

- **Shortness of breath**

Action I take: balance breathing, lay down, stress control through meditation. Difficulty in breathing may very well be the first symptom I experienced. A symptom I could not ignore on a golf course. Mark it up to excessive sunlight, or having a long day. I am convinced the shortness of breath for me is MS related. What could I do about it? I could use my balanced breathing technique (pranayama). Meditate and even try to walk it off. This "grasping for a breath does go away after I apply some form of healing technique. Also, this shortness of breath comes and goes in varying degrees. This does not have to be stress related. I can be grasping for air for no reason at all. Then this symptom will go away for months.

- **Ringing ears**

Action I take: Balance breathing, meditation. I live with varying degrees of ear ringing daily.

I make note of this situation because in the past the tinnitus was real strong. This is sometimes called "Head Noise". I did look into the causes and what I could do about it. What I learned conditions such as Menieres disease seems to be even worse. My ear ringing is manageable on a daily basis. Some days are worse than others. Is this MS related? I believe so. Come to think about it, again, fatigue may play a role in the ear ringing. Early on I had my doctor clean my ears. No help. Wax or no wax they still ring. But having my ears cleaned sure felt good!

Have I found a way to abate the symptom? Meditation works at least for awhile.

- **Overheating**

Action I take: Rest, ice water, icepack behind neck, and on forehead. Lay down.

I have spent fifteen years in Hawaii. Five of those years with a confirmed diagnosis of MS on my chart. Fortunately I carry very little body fat. I can say the low fat diet that *Dr. Swank* and others talk about is extremely important in keeping my weight balanced. Extra body weight will not help the heat issue. I wear a hat and minimize sun exposure. I just try to be careful. The heat will make my gait wider and more wobbly. Sometimes light headed, but I know how to avoid the symptoms so I do. A quick way to diminish any symptom in the heat is for me to put a pack of ice on the neck and top of head and lay down. There may be relief in just a few minutes.

Tools for Management of MS Symptoms

1. Meditation

2. Balanced breathing

3. Rest and sleep

4. Sesame oil massage

5. Protein for fuel

6. Vitamins

7. Herbs

8. Stretching

9. Walking

10. Weight Lifting

11. Reading Inspiring Books

12. Affirmations

13. Keep a journal active

14. Never give up

15. Wheatgrass

16. Brush teeth

17. Tongue scraping

This list has taken years of trial and error to compile. This is by no means a recommendation to anyone. This is now my toolbox. Some of these tools may prove to be of little or no help for you. This is a good place for you to start your own toolbox and discover what works best for you. Please remember, it is up to you to document your daily journal so you can track your progress. A concerned friend or relative may tell you about an herb they feel might help you. You may see an article in a magazine about visualization techniques. If you decide to follow through with these tips write them down. Research them. You will have your own list. From B12 vitamin sublingual's dissolved under the tongue to meditation, *you* are in control. Keep track in a journal with a timeline of how each product or technique works or did not work in your particular situation. With a journal and including dates you will have a better idea if something is working for you or not. Another excellent outcome of keeping a journal is having the ability to refer back to your own writings concerning a particular issue you may find yourself dealing with in the future. Really, if I had not been keeping a journal all these years, I would not be able to write this book. My mind is full of healing techniques I have used. To put them on paper and present them to you would be impossible without my journals.

1. Meditation. I was fortunate to be taught Transcendental Meditation or TM by my Medical Doctor, *Dr. Douwe Rienstra*. How about this for a great asset and healer? I have also followed meditation techniques from books by *Dr. Chopra* and *Dr. Andrew Weil*. Yes, it is great to learn from a TM teacher like I did, but the main theme here is to learn and begin meditation immediately. You can begin right now by sitting quietly, close your eyes and follow each breath with your mind. Visualize the oxygen entering your body and leaving your body. You will experience a calming feeling. Practice this for twenty minutes twice a day. Write this down in your journal.

2. Balanced Breathing. "Pranayama" is a simple and extremely rewarding technique to practice immediately. I refer again to *Dr. Chopra's* book *"Perfect Health"*. *Dr. Chopra* speaks of balance breathing in this wonderful book. This technique takes only a few minutes to learn. My first experience with meditation improved my breathing immediately. Healing is balance. I cannot over emphasize this moment in my experience with MS. Using breathing techniques entering into meditation resulted in my ability to relax the symptoms

as they were thrown at me, and balance my own controls. The discomfort of symptoms at this time is impossible to ignore. I have become better at dealing with the symptoms. One step at a time. Eastern medicine philosophy is proficient at this. In America we are used to the quick fix. But Multiple Sclerosis has no quick fix.

3. Rest and sleep. Often times I will balance my breathing, meditate and fall asleep. I will spend a half hour to an hour with these techniques. If I fall asleep for a longer period of time, this becomes a healing opportunity.

4. Sesame oil massage. In 1991 I experienced a major breakthrough in my healing the day I gave myself the first sesame oil massage. Each massage only uses a couple tablespoons of warm sesame or coconut oil. After applying you merely wipe off the excess oil with a paper towel, then shower. Again, my great medical doctor, *Dr. Rienstra* recommended this technique to me and certainly other patients. *Dr. Chopra* in his book *"Perfect Health"* shows this technique. I remember taking an incredible deep breath with my first sesame oil massage. To breathe is to heal. I have to say when you search for a medical doctor, search for a doctor that is skilled and comfortable with alternative approaches and Western medicine. With *Dr. Rienstra* I found complete authenticity in his practice. *Dr. Rienstra* attempts to do all he can to help his patients help themselves. In your search for a medical doctor I would highly recommend one that embodies the knowledge of Western and Eastern medicine. There are more and more physicians with these abilities if you do the research. My first experience with sesame oil massage in 1991 came with a host of new sensations. Fourteen years later I remember taking that first tablespoon of heated oil in my palm and pouring this over my head. Beginning to lightly massage this oil into my hair and scalp and onto the joints and lymph nodes. This immediately made me take a deep breath. This was a natural process of relief through inhaling oxygen. Remember to breathe is to heal.

5. Protein for fuel. Every morning for breakfast I have a soy protein drink in a glass of vanilla soy milk. I use a product called "Natures Life Pro 96" soy protein. However, I do add some "Natures Plus" soy protein powder on occasion for variety. When I am at Mom and Dad's house I will also have a bowl of oatmeal topped with vanilla soy milk and a little honey for sweetener. In between meals I always have lots of nuts and boiled eggs around. I avoid "running out of gas" with my diet. I do not overeat but I avoid being famished. Balance.

6. Vitamins. See chapter 6

7. Herbs. See chapter 6

8. Stretching and exercises. See chapter 8. I limit my exercises to fifteen to thirty minutes every morning; I do not overdo this because I can become ill with MS symptoms.

9. Walking. I have continued to make it a requirement to walk every day. Yes, during the first throes of MS I walked after every meal, which was incredibly important because my bowels were so affected. Rain or shine I walk a half hour after dinner. My digestive system appreciates this. Always.

10. Weight lifting. See chapter 8. I have a set of free weights I have used off and on through the years. Beginning with two pound dumbbells.

11. Read inspiring books and research MS. I read lots of books and articles, every day mostly about health.

12. Affirmations. This is a daily routine. Prayers under my breath. Giving thanks daily to God. Prayer is a 'whole brain' experience that aligns your spiritual being with your physical being.

13. Keep a journal active. Sometimes my journals are full day after day. Other days I draw a blank. If symptoms are bothersome, remember your journal. Write in it. You will be glad you did.

14. Never give up. The word "quit" is not in the vocabulary of this book. Dr. Chopra's books are full of reasons why you should never give up.

15. Wheatgrass. *"The Wheatgrass book"* by *Ann Wigmore* and published by Avery books, convinced me to cultivate and grow wheatgrass. Three years and 1000 trays of wheatgrass later I am happy I did.

16. Brush Teeth. I wake up and first thing, I brush my teeth with a little baking soda. I will then scrape my tongue. After every meal I brush my teeth. After drinking coffee I brush my teeth.

17. Tongue scraping. Every morning with my first tooth brushing I scrape my tongue. This is an Ayurvedic health rule. The result is that "ama" is removed from your tongue. Digestion begins in your mouth. Most health food stores have tongue scrapers. A company called "Dr. Tung" is a readily available brand.

Vitamins, Herbs, Omega - Three Oils I Rely on Today

This list of daily supplements I take has changed many times over the years. I expect you will see this in your own diary as you begin to map out the present and future. Your medical doctor should be able to suggest vitamins, proteins, and herbs etc. for your daily regimen. Also, refer to Ann Boroch's book "Healing Multiple Sclerosis" for additional information. Beyond my own research I have relied on a friend who has been in the health industry for over thirty years. I graduated from High School with John Thoreson in 1968. John is instrumental in my decisions. I rely on his expertise. At this time I am taking the following supplements.

1. Seriphos: By T.E. Neesby www.amazon.com/t-e-neesby.seriphos. An important supplement for the central nervous system. I have taken Seriphos for ten years. Ask your doctor about this extremely important supplement.

2. Multivitamin: I purchase at the heal food store I work at.

3. Fish Oil or Cod Liver Oil: Nordic Naturals, Carlson Labs, or Pharmax brands. Follow directions on label.

4. Acidopholis: That contains both bifidobacterium and lactobacillus strains. Three billion and above, cells per capsule. Follow directions on label.

5. Vitamin C: In powder form. 5,000 mg. per day or to bowel tolerance.

6. Vitamin E: d-alpha tocopheryl sucinate 400 i.e. follow directions on label.

7. Vitamin D3: 1000 i.e. follow directions on label. Ask your doctor.

8. CoQ10: 90-150 mg. Follow your doctors recommendations.

Herb combinations:

9. Memoran: An Ayurvedic combination from Ayush Herbs. www.ayush.com. Ask your doctor. Follow directions on label.

10. Ashwaganda: An Ayurvedic herb from Ayush Herbs. www.ayush.com. Follow directions on label.

11. Amla Plex: by Ayush herbs. www.ayush.com. Follow directions on label.

12. Eyebright: Health food stores. Follow directions on label.

Over the last fourteen years I have also used the following products. Yes, I have healed. A lot. However, please take the time to research websites, read books on referrals for other vitamins and herbs that help people with MS. I do not profess to know it all! For more information, contact your doctor and do your own research.

1. Sunrider herb combination (www.sunrider.com) known as "Quinary" plus Top, Joi, Ese., Nuplus, and Calli beverage.

2. Pycnogenol

3. Essiac tea

4. B12 sublinguals

5. Spirulina

6. Evening primrose oil

7. Flax oil

8. MSM (methylsulfonymethane)

9. Calms forte

10. Lecithin granuals

Foods I Rely on

As my diet changed in preparation for a life with MS, food became simpler and actually more creative. Early in my healing I really concentrated on avoiding processed foods containing sugar. Even too much fruit was noticeable. Once I read "The Yeast Connection" and practiced the elimination of Candida I balanced my system. I can have an occasional homemade piece of pie with no problem. Fruit no problem. Yes, I accept simple foods. I enjoy foods that make me feel good! Food is fuel. I do not overeat. I eat in restaurants infrequently. I begin every morning with two 8oz. glasses of filtered water. This is also the time I take my vitamin "Seriphos" and often times some vitamin C in the water. Right after this I will spend 20 minutes sitting quietly and practicing meditation. I will also do a fifteen to thirty minute routine of stretching and exercise. Then I will mix an 8oz. glass of vanilla soy milk with a scoop of "Natures Life Pro 96" soy protein or comparable protein. I will take my morning vitamins at this time. Plus an acidophilus supplement. After this, I will enjoy a double shot of espresso with hot water. Within 2 hours I will have a boiled egg with a little mustard, and a handful of nuts of any kind.

For lunch I will steam a vegetable, open a can of water packed tuna fish and mix with mayonnaise, chopped dill or sweet pickles, a little mustard, ground pepper, etc. I will pile this tuna fish on top of the steamed vegetables. A sliced fruit is also a regular on my table. Potato chips if I have them. Candy and Malcolm, two of my six cats like potato chips.

A three p.m. snack I may have another boiled egg, nuts, soy protein drink, etc. I avoid getting too hungry. Meditation before dinner is also perfect timing. Dinner can mimic lunch. There are wonderful recipes in just about every cookbook that can be adapted to fit a non-dairy, low saturated fat diet. I love to bake and like to cook but I do not focus on this at this time. Food is fuel to live comfortably and heal.

My diet:

1. Filtered water

2. Natures Life Pro 96 soy protein

3. Vanilla soy milk (Kirkland brand – Costco)

4. Boiled, poached, fried (with extra virgin olive oil) egg, etc.

5. Almonds, cashews, sunflower seeds, pumpkin seeds, macadamia nuts, pecans.

6. Flourless bread or Ezekial 4.9 (maybe 4 slices a week)

7. Jewel yams, squash of all kinds - steamed.

8. Broccoli

9. Red skinned potatoes

10. Carrots

11. Kale

12. Miso

13. Tahini

14. Fresh fish

15. Water packed albacore tuna (Kirkland brand if available)

16. Kipper snacks (smoked herring filets)

17. Apples

18. Oranges

19. Pineapple

20. Bananas

21 Potato chips! (Non-hydrogenated oil)

22. Catsup (a brand like Westbrae) no high fructose corn syrup

23. Mustard

24. Soy sauce

25. Mayonnaise

26. Dill pickles

27. Sweet pickles occasionally

28. Olives of all varieties

29. Canned vegetable soup on occasion. Then I embellish the tomato based soup.

Exercise and Stretching
I Rely on

I have read countless books on MS. Other people's beginnings, diagnosis, life changes. Moderation in exercise seems to be the healthiest avenue. When I over did my exercise routine, I would increase symptoms. I met a Navy Seal soldier early in my diagnosis. This young man was in a wheel chair. I can only imagine the strenuous training he went through. Was this healthy? There are books on the shelf now with women who exercised 2 hours a day as a routine. Now they are dealing with MS. Can we "physically" tax our bodies and minds to such an extreme that MS is awakened?

Balanced breathing begins my exercise. Illustrated in *"Perfect Health"* by *Dr Deepak Chopra.* 30 to 95 sit ups daily.

One to ten Yoga Sun Salutes every day. Illustrated in many books on yoga and healing to include *"Perfect Health"* by *Dr. Deepak Chopra.*

Weight lifting with free weights. Illustrated in many books to include *Bill Pearls* book *"Getting Stronger".* Light weights in moderation.

Walking after dinner nightly – approximately thirty minutes – for digestion. Balance. When I was in the throes of MS I walked after every meal at least fifteen minutes. My digestion was so hampered in the beginning, I needed this routine. Just walking 30 minutes nightly is 1.5 miles on my route. Thirty days in a row with this walk I have accomplished 45 miles of walking for the month after dinner!

Patrick as a person
growing up

Laying claim to one's self on paper in book form is not like filling out an application for employment or paperwork to buy a car. No. There is some stumbling to begin with. Perhaps the lack of finding my life that interesting or different. But anyone that has lived on this planet for fifty-four years including myself has something to write about besides a job application.

Growing up in an idealic environment with wonderful parents, sisters and home on a small town farm, who could ask for more? I finished high school in 1968 and attended a four year college in the fall. With absolutely no idea what I wanted to do with myself I grew my hair long and joined the rest of the "counter culture" and all the trappings of the days. I should not be excluded from any of the name calling for those days as my Mom would mention more than once over the next twenty years. Surviving the first ten years of learning out of high school as a college drop-out was "a trip" as many of us will attest to in the early seventies.

I was always "type A" ambitious. I held all sorts of jobs. Logger, tree trimmer, roofer, remote terminal typist, and teletype operator. With never a hint towards a looming disease in my future. Or was there?

I continued to re-analyze my childhood nervousness which showed me pulling all my eye lashes out of my eye lids during grade school, biting the inside of my cheeks raw through high school to an extremely nervous stomach before most every class. This included gym. Does this sound familiar? So bothersome at times my mother hauled me to the doctor to check on my nervous stomach. The doctor had me drink heavy pink liquid called barium before a couple of the office visits. So the doctor could have a look at my stomach and most parts in between. Only to have no definitive answers. Yes, this is a clue. Something has got to give in the physical and mental future.

During 1978 while being employed as a radio dispatcher for the County Sheriff's Department, I bought a donut shop in a little town in Eastern Washington. I had always been interested in baking. I helped my Mom bake pies and cut in the butter and Crisco (now we know about hydrogenated and trans fats!). Never shying away from something new, I found myself waking at three a.m. six days a week to bake bread and deep fry donuts at my new bakery. As a side note, I did not eat fried donuts. My days as a free spirit had taught me about fried foods and the importance of whole wheat, etc. So donuts were not a part of my diet. My job as a dispatcher was a night job so I had no problem working twelve hour days at the bakery until my relief would show up at 3:00 p.m.

Thousands of donuts and thousands of loaves of bread later I met my wife Kim Onette Starr, an artist, in 1980. Meeting Kim became another chapter in my life. I went from deep frying donuts and baking bread in Eastern Washington to living on the Big Island of Hawaii running Kim Starr Gallery for nine years. One would think living in my early thirties in the Hawaiian Islands running an art gallery and married to a very beautiful and accomplished artist, any nervousness as a kid would disappear as an adult. I should just grow out of nervousness like a pair of pants? This does not appear to be the case concerning the central nervous system. I think of myself as an energetic person. My central nervous system wound tight as a child to the present.

To avoid the recollection of additional years in any more of a descriptive nature, I will refer you to the cover of this book, a Kim Starr oil painting. This work of art seemed appropriate for the title *"Bouncing Back"*.

Yet in this sunshine world some strange things were afoot that only in retrospection.....would begin to add up. Mangoes as they fell from the tree, causing loud clanging sounds on our tin roofed house. Lack of sound sleep, difficulty in lining up to a golf ball on a golf course, picking up a pen off the desk at my office to slurred speech, to the ominous gait wobbles that came and went. Time passed. Then a startling morning wakeup call of a symptom (I will talk more about that later in Chapter ten).

My MS Journey

Note: Readers of this book may want to skip this chapter and chapter fourteen. This was important to me and certainly points out my "gradual" climb out of some of the traumas of life through the eyes of someone living with Multiple Sclerosis. That said, you can always go back and read "my MS journey" and "timeline" once you begin your own journals and formulate your own program to live with MS.

September 3, 1990, I woke up frightened out of my mind! My journal, my life with MS pretty much started at this time. In fact, it was fourteen years ago I woke up to a brilliant morning. Unfortunately the brilliance struck me as pulsating flashes in my field of vision but no sight and no balance. I struggled out of bed, reeled around and just dropped to the bedroom floor. It was violent. This was my first major exacerbation with MS, although at the time, I had no idea what was happening. I was just completely disoriented. Four doctors, many tests, and five weeks later came the diagnosis of Multiple Sclerosis. Now I was really scared! I had no idea what MS was but I was relieved I didn't have a brain tumor. No one said "Keep a journal Pat, it will give you much needed control, make you responsible to your circumstances, it will become a refuge, and remarkably it can function as an irreplaceable guide." Yet, on that day I dusted off an old journal and made and entry, September 03, 1990… and started writing. I didn't realize it then just how powerful a tool this journal would become. I will tell you again, "keep a journal" for these very reasons. Start one today.

When I was diagnosed the first doctor was pessimistic. No answers were offered to my questions. I felt lost, distraught, and out of control. The doctors in 1990 had no disease modifying drugs approved by the FDA for MS to recommend, and had there been, my story may well have turned out differently. Since then I have never taken disease modifying drugs (there are currently four) although this choice to "just say no" to drugs has been mine, not my doctors. I had to find some way to gain a sense of hope, to regain some sense of control in my life, and to get well.

Now, after living with MS for fourteen years, I still have MS. Some symptoms still come and go daily, yet I'm doing it without drugs or wheelchairs. I want everyone, especially with MS, who picks up this book to be encouraged to lay a claim to being well again and take control of their own health. You are the one who stands to benefit. How can you make this happen? Of the many questions I have asked over the course of the past fourteen years living with MS what I offer you in this book would have been of great help when I was first diagnosed. Now you can start with fundamental things to do (see chapter two) which I have found to be positive. I can prioritize actions to take and things to change that have the biggest positive effect in helping to overcome the debilitating symptoms of MS. Remember, I am only speaking for myself through my experience in living with MS. All fellow MS'rs will create their own path through diagnosis and life with Multiple Sclerosis. Take control NOW.

A word about the present disease modifying drugs:

*At the present time they must be injected. Although manufacturers are working on oral versions.

* Side effects are usually manageable.

* Their overall effectiveness is modest.

* They are expensive.

Reconsider for a moment here the recommendation of *Dr. Swank's*, saying if you start to take responsibility for your life with MS and begin to make the suggested lifestyle and dietary changes now you can live a happier, healthier life. The earlier in the disease process you make the positive changes he says the more profound. Now that sounds good! Believe me; I am so glad I found a great doctor. It is one of the first things to do in my "most important things to do" list. We need "good medicine" and so it is easy to become frustrated and disheartened when our choices are confined to the products offered in a drug store.

The day I was diagnosed with Multiple Sclerosis, I began reading about MS and formulating my own opinions on living with MS. Since this was exactly what I was now facing minute by minute. My reading was not exclusively set to the *National Multiple Sclerosis Society* recommended readings. Actually, I began borrowing books from my medical doctor's office. *Dr. Rienstra* started me on the path to heal. I shall be ever grateful for his approach to medicine. *Dr Rienstra* became a hero in my eyes. How often do you look in a doctor's office and see a "lending library" of books such as written by *Dr. Chopra* and others?

Why did I begin a journal in the first place? This is one question in September of 1990, I did not have an answer for. I had tried writing in a journal before but with no staying power. This time I just wrote in a notebook. I was physically and mentally distraught and in trouble trying to understand these rapid changes. The journal may have been my own way of dealing with how I felt. A temporary relief from a symptom? Things were not working the way they should physically. I was scared. I felt rotten. What will Kim do? What will my parents think? What about our art gallery business? Our future plans?

My first "self-recorded" in a journal exacerbation was a doozy! This one got my attention. The morning I awakened and immediately realized I could not see anything. Then strobes of wiry colors showed up after a minute or so. I dropped to the floor grabbing for the side of the bed. After a few minutes, I gained my composure and now blurred vision followed. However, the dizziness remained for the uneven walk to the bathroom. Boy oh boy, what was that?! I realized the bathroom was waiting for me. I had lost my bowel control. This attack or "exacerbation" really started my writing in a journal. My life has been different ever since. At the age of forty there were some things I began to learn about health that are with me today. The Multiple Sclerosis diagnosis has not been a quick study for me. I have been reading and learning ever since. However, I did have a great thirst to get my life back to "normal" as soon as possible. In September 1990 I did not realize that "normal" was something I would strive for only to find normal is always going to be a little out of reach from now on.

How on earth can someone live like this? Now I can tell you how I go about life with MS. To stick with this journal since 1990 for no reason – maybe the reason has now presented itself. I have not discovered the fountain of youth for MS patients. Actually, Dr Swank, Dr Deepak Chopra, John Pageler, Ann Boroch and others have already championed techniques to help us live with MS. To me, this is the only way to live day to day. Kim asks me how I can be so disciplined with diet and exercise. I have said over and over again, I really have no choice. To me, I am taking the only path to living with MS.

Growing up as a kid we tend to be accustomed to having someone else such as a trusted medical doctor to fix everything. Sorry, not this time. If there is such a thing as a "textbook" case of MS, I probably fit in this category. I consulted four different doctors before a definitive Multiple Sclerosis diagnosis. This diagnosis came from neurologists as a result of an MRI scan. With the revelation of the diagnosis comes the thinking back part for all of us with MS. When did the first symptom appear? The answer for me would be on a golf course. I could not line up the ball and the head of the club. I was way off. This never happened until now. The year was 1983; I was thirty-three years old at the time. Frustrated, I walked off the course. I thought I was probably just coming down with the flu or a cold or something. Nothing serious. I was too young for serious. Golf was not a game I played very often so I do not remember a problem like this before or after this incident.

Three years later in 1986 as I sat in my office at an art gallery Kim and I owned on the Kona side of the Big Island of Hawaii I was surprised with "slurred speech." This was another totally new experience for me. My speech was sounding really weird. A slow motion in speech. I attempted to mask the speech at the gallery and around Kim. A week passed and speech was back to normal. Looking back I also remember my inability to pick up a pen. I would put my hand down to pick up a pen and I would be an inch and a half off. What's this I thought? This affliction lasted a few days and went away. In hindsight, this was another exacerbation. Maybe no long lasting brain scars but still an exacerbation.

One more incident, as I look back sometime in 1989, I was having a very difficult time sleeping. So bad that I consulted a physician. A routine physical examination and tests were done. Nothing significant showed. But then, in my own searching, I came up with the realization that mangos falling off a tree directly over the bedroom roof must be keeping me from sleeping through the night. When the mango season ended, sleep returned.

Now, in 2004, I question this mango dropping diagnosis seriously enough for me to consult a doctor. Mangos hitting a tin roof? Probably not the reason for my sleep interruption. Exacerbation more likely. Since my diagnosis I found myself living all the emotions, physical changes and overall heightened awareness of life and mind.

This book has in a way taken the same amount of years to write. My diary entries can be as small as a sentence in a week with no mention of health issues to a couple of pages of a day fraught with symptoms and emotions, to gaps of months with no writing at all. For anyone who has or is going through the physical realm of MS has all experienced what the medical field calls an "exacerbation." I have experienced sight difficulties, vertigo, loss of balance, slurred speech, ear ringing, numbness, fatigue, wide gait, etc. Take your pick. One with MS also has a heightened ability to view a change no matter how insignificant as a part of an exacerbation.

Early in my balancing act of healing, I found the analogy "two steps forward, one step back" quite accurate, but anyone with MS knows the duration of the steps back are omnipresent and impossible to ignore. No timeline to follow.

Certain symptoms can be with me for days, weeks, months on end with little change. This is really where I had to reach into my book of tools and convince myself I should level out. There were no drugs to grab hold of. Dealing with symptoms at least during the first five years was day by day. Practice, Practice, Practice.

For the most part I lead my life the same as I led my life in 1970 and 1980. I am wild with ideas at fifty four years of age just like I have always been. I am blessed with a wonderful partner in Kim, my wife of twenty-two plus years, six cats, my Mom and Dad and two sisters. Age found me growing up in a real life setting not unlike the television show "Leave it to Beaver." My parents taught me the value of a positive self worth. I am finding this "self worth" to be one of the tools of my MS healing tool box. When I was in my 20's and formulating life as I saw it, I was not slowing down to smell the roses. Growing up in a functional family environment is definitely a positive tool in my tool box. The way I approach new ideas and challenges is "I can." This attitude came early on in my childhood. My parents were instrumental in teaching me the value of self worth. I have a good friend who was diagnosed with MS after me and is not walking anymore unfortunately. Danny's upbringing did not embody the nurturing value of positive thinking I experienced.

This mental tool in the healing tool box is of great value. Books can help. From *Deepak Chopra* to *Norman Vincent Peale,* the enhancement of positive thinking as a useable tool is paramount. There are no short cuts in the work that needs to be done when building self esteem from books. This is a daily if not an hourly exercise. Added stress of MS makes the challenge even more difficult. To achieve balance to counteract MS, the tools of self worth must be added. No matter what it takes. No matter how many prayers, how many positive affirmations an hour you repeat you must continue.

Dr. Douwe Rienstra, my primary care physician in Port Townsend, Washington, recommended that I read "Creating Health" by *Dr. Chopra.* I found such encouraging help in *Chopra's* writing, which I read pages over and over again. More books by *Dr. Chopra* as *"Quantum Healing"* and *"Perfect*

Health" were added to my healing toolbox. You can literally help change physical situations via mental exercise. You can better your present situation? You do not have to feel rotten all the time. I felt optimistic for the first time since diagnosis. There is help. I will add books to my tool box to heal.

Feeling rotten with a neurological imbalance is being uncomfortable from the skin inward. Feeling the malaise of other MS symptoms is constant. Fatigue being a result that is hard to ignore and accept. This neurological cocktail of physical and emotional symptoms stayed with me the first time for three years. I had tried to lead a normal life but this was impossible with MS. Just too many symptoms with no warning of change in the future. From these early years I learned that every day brought differences in my physical being, my mental being and my emotional being. I kept writing enough in my journal to track my life with MS. I spent countless hours reading about Multiple Sclerosis. I read *Dr. Deepak Chopra* books, *"Creating Health"* and *"Quantum Healing"* over and over again.

Finding My Way

In March of 1991, a friend of mine called me in Port Townsend, Washington, where I was living at the time. Her name is *Dinah Kunitake*. Dinah had heard of my battles with MS. Dinah thought she had a combination of herbs that would benefit me. She took it upon herself to contact me. To reach out. I care very deeply for Dinah to this day. I really appreciated the contact.

The herbs came from a mail order company called Sunrider. Dinah sent me a combination of herbs she felt would be beneficial plus information on the herbs. At this particular time, my energy had been drained. My central nervous system was out of balance. I felt uncomfortable in my own skin with little relief. Even trying to watch television was impossible. The TV rattled my nervous system too much.

I remember going to the movies. I spent the whole length of the movie in the lobby not watching the movie, "Dances with Wolves." I could not handle the noise and the flash of the movie screen at all. My only comfort zone that winter became walking by myself rain or snow and praying to heal. This is when I came up with my own combination of words to recite.

"I give my mind and body the tools, the time and the desire to heal."

I did however intermix the "Lord's Prayer" during those walks. This addition of prayer was from growing up Catholic and going to church every Sunday. I said these words thousands and thousands of times while walking and sitting. Often times on the side of a road with the rain pouring down upon me. No relief. I would walk the roads and feel the tears stream down my face uncontrollably. I was a mess. I often asked myself how could I be married to such a beautiful and perfect person, have so much to live for and be affected with this uncontrollable disease?

My first experience with my newly arrived bottle of herbs from my friend was a positive one. I took the combination called quinary with breakfast. I am not sure what specific feeling I had but within the hour I asked Kim if she would like to play catch with a baseball. Kim and I played catch in the backyard. This was a huge change from the previous twenty-four hours. Until that moment I had only scattered relief from the symptoms. I was a neurological mess. I was coping through life. That evening I did not take the herbs. I felt if I could feel this different I better not take the recommended dose three times a day. I had better take it slowly. I was not sure I could sleep, I felt so different.

From the time of diagnosis through the first three years of healing I had relied on a prescription drug called Ativan to help me relax and sleep. My most significant exacerbation came with an awakening without sight, just strobing colors, no balance, and loss of bowel control all at once. From then on I was afraid to go to bed in fear I would wake like that again. Going to bed reading something positive, ½ of an Ativan and I would be able to sleep. In the morning I would awaken, yes, even refreshed. But within fifteen minutes of what I call the "yuks" which includes vertigo would appear again. At the beginning of taking the Sunrider herbs, around six months after the MS diagnosis, I had my first fifteen minutes of "relief" when I first awakened in the morning. I actually felt "normal" for fifteen minutes a day. This may not sound like much but the six months before then I did not find a minute of "normalcy" while awake. These fifteen minutes became a goal and target for me. The previous six months was consumed with praying, reading and walking to try and ignore the never ending "yuks." The morning fifteen minutes of normalcy was a welcomed relief and goal. I wanted to be better. I wanted to stretch those fifteen minutes to longer. Why not?

Dr. Chopra in *"Creating Health"* and *"Quantum Healing"* wrote about how man is not as solid as a sculpture but instead we are changing constantly. Like a flowing river. The basis of regeneration. I was in close contact with *Dr. Rienstra.* He introduced Kim and me to Transcendental Meditation. *Dr. Rienstra* believed TM would be excellent for everyone. *Dr. Chopra* has written much about meditation. The technique was taught by *Dr. Rienstra* in his clinic in Port Townsend. Can you imagine being so fortunate to have your medical doctor so practiced in other forms of medicine to be able to offer an alternative approach to Western medicine when he feels an alternate approach could be beneficial? Especially in a long term treatment of a major disease. What an opportunity.

The classes were at night. I was so tired by that time I was fraught with MS symptoms my head would be resting on Kim's shoulder during the classes. Over the two weeks we had learned about the basics of Transcendental Meditation and we were ready to meditate on our own. Dr. Rienstra suggested a morning meditation before breakfast and an evening meditation before dinner. Dr. Rienstra also began teaching us a very simple technique called balanced breathing. This is known as "pranayama" in Ayurvedic medicine. An excellent explanation with illustrations may be found on page 300 and 301 of "Perfect Health" by Dr. Chopra.

Kim and I practiced meditation with dedication. My fifteen minutes of normalcy per day became thirty-five minutes. I began to have an hour in the morning symptom free. I was beginning to experience something close to "normalcy" except for lack of bowel control, vertigo and balance. I did stay away from climbing ladders. The morning relief from the "yuks" was helping me learn and experiment with exercise. I would pick up a set of dumbbells and follow a book titled *"Getting Stronger"* by *Bill Pearl* on weight lifting. I would balance my breathing and complete a few sun salutes. I experimented with foods to see how they made me feel. My bowels were sensitive and reacted like a "hair triggered" gun. If I ate a little too much I would be faced with diarrhea. Following the diarrhea was a bout of faintness. During the first six months this was happening all the time. I learned to map out in my mind the closest bathroom available in any instance. Around the eighth month time frame, Kim and I drove to Roseburg, Oregon. We were investigating a move to a sunnier climate but still on the West Coast. We had lived on the Big Island of Hawaii since 1981 but at this time in 1990 we felt the need to stay on the West Coast. Of course moving takes money and we really had none. We had a small house payment and equity in our home in Port Townsend.

The potential move would take us away from our present house location which unfortunately loomed awfully close to a paper mill. This environment was not a good place to live while trying to heal from MS or any type of serious disease. We chose Roseburg, Oregon, four hundred miles south and inland. Housing prices were very reasonable. We could afford to purchase a house in Roseburg and at the same time be that much closer to warmer weather. While staying at a hotel in Roseburg, Kim and I ordered lunch at the adjoining restaurant. I distinctly remember ordering vegetables with a cheese sauce. Within the hour I could not stay away from the toilet. My bowels were in control of me. What a night.

The next day I was wasted for the trip back to Port Townsend. Just about that time I had come across a small paperback book titled *"New Hope Real Help for People with MS"* by *John Pageler*. John touted *"No Dairy"* period! Well, I read those words and that was an eye opener. I hadn't even seen *"The Multiple Sclerosis Diet Book"* by *Dr. Roy Swank*. From that day forward, *no dairy for me*. I had stopped eating red meat, chicken, turkey etc. in 1974. I was used to eating cheese for protein on everything I could put it on. Or just by itself. I also grew up with a never ending ice cream bowl. The three gallon tubs of Neapolitan ice cream were readily available. Adulthood and a move to Hawaii in 1981 brought Haagen-Dazs ice cream to my table. Dairy had always been a big part of my diet. My physical frame showed little body fat. I have always been thin. I could eat all the fat and dairy I wanted. Now this! MS. I shall never eat ice cream again. No cheese cake. I had no problem adjusting. I wanted to give myself all the opportunity to heal.

With the wonderful writing of *John Pageler* followed by the "no more dairy" wake up call in Roseburg, I experienced another change in my physical symptoms. Eliminating dairy from my diet showed a positive side to my bowel control almost immediately. To this day I am well aware of potential bathroom sights. But now I have my control back so I can actually plan a bathroom visit instead of a hurried visit. For anyone with MS they can certainly relate. Once I removed dairy from my diet, I experienced another milestone in healing. I needed to address the loss of dairy protein and specifically cheese as a protein source for convenience. After all, cheese goes with just about anything, and is great tasting by itself!! And how convenient! Give it up I say! The daily protein loss was apparent. I felt this loss in my ability to think, energy, and even balance. Protein to me, with little or no physical reserves is a number one requirement in my diet.

A wonderful protein source I quickly assimilated was eggs. As a boy growing up I was responsible for the care of 50 white leghorn chickens. I had a weekly egg route and my own rubber stamp for the cartons. "Pat's Farm Fresh Eggs". A boiled egg to this day can be a savior. I will have boiled eggs in the car with any outing over an hour long. For a walk, I will take a boiled egg along. Nothing fancy. Deviled eggs are great, but just a boiled egg in my pocket is adequate. The eggs are rarely returned to the refrigerator. In my search for protein sources, I experimented with soy products. I began my search with a soy protein and vanilla soy milk every morning. I could feel the nutrition entering my system within a few minutes. Tuna fish is also a quick protein supplement. Kim will also steam organic broccoli, kale and all sorts of vegetables. The accomplishment of having no symptoms in the first fifteen minutes of the day opposed to no symptoms before ten in the morning seems to be the result of the combination for me.

The first three years were spent experimenting with combinations of foods and vitamins that worked for me. You will need to experiment as I did. Only time will tell if you are on the right track. Certain foods as I entered them into my routine immediately did not work. Overeating anything is a mistake. I remember asking *Dr. Rienstra* one time if I could improve my condition. He answered abruptly what if you don't improve? This answer with a question really caught me off guard. I went home without the comfort of the answer I wanted to hear. After revisiting this question years later I felt *Dr. Rienstra* was preparing me for the unknown future living with MS. However, I was convinced I was making a difference in the changes I was making.

Another suggestion *Dr. Rienstra* made was concerning shopping at the grocery store. Stay in the outer isles. Stay away from the packaged foods. What about peanut butter as a protein source I asked? Almond butter he answered.

During the early years I was reading everything I could about MS and any subjects on health. During this time I came across the *"Wheatgrass Book"* by *Anne Wigmore*. She convinced me to start cultivating the tender grass. Using a wheatgrass squeezer to extract the rich chlorophyll. I would harvest and squeeze a tray of wheatgrass a day. Twice a day I would drink a shot glass full of chlorophyll. This amounted to six fluid ounces of chlorophyll per tray. The germination period from seed to harvest is ten days. This required eighteen trays of wheatgrass in various stages of growth at all times. This is a very potent tasting drink and may take some time to acquire a taste for. I would also mix the wheatgrass with fresh squeezed carrot, apple and ginger juice. My MS symptoms were almost always present but I could feel healing. Was it the daily ingestion of wheatgrass that made a difference? I will never know for sure. The wheatgrass costs pennies to grow per shot. I did reduce my intake of Sunrider herbs. My herb bill definitely dropped off. The "yuks" had diminished but other symptoms became more prevalent. Some fatigue was expected by two to three in the afternoon every day. Vertigo was a daily experience with me in varying degrees. I began having mornings with fewer bowel issues and less fatigue. It is possible this increased my awareness of vertigo coupled with a "floating feeling." A paper mill that loomed below the cliff in our backyard in Port Townsend may have been emitting something from its huge smoke stacks that was affecting my nervous system.

During the first three years of healing, meditation, herbs, wheatgrass, yoga sun salutes, diet changes, etc. I kept my diary going, however sketchy it was. It identified highs and lows in my physical dilemma. Two steps forward, one step backward. I tried to keep a positive outlook.

In 1994, I was asked by a friend if I would be interested in working in a health food store if he bought the store. In fact, he was only going to purchase the business if I would agree to work in the store. We reached a one year agreement. I would have the ability to work the hours that fit me and also buy all herbs, books, vitamins, etc. at cost. This was another step and positive situation in my healing. We were taking over a failing health food store with a juice bar. But Charlie, the new owner, nor I ever had a second thought about its potential success. It would be up to us to make the business work and grow. I had access to all sorts of new products at cost. I could order any books for sale for the store. This became a very positive situation for me. I was taking home literature on vitamins and minerals and herbs daily. Studying health issues from A to Z. Not just Multiple Sclerosis. From *COQ10* to *Acidopholis* to *Spirulina*, I learned as much as I could about the products. I did have a goal to try to lower my herb bill as much as possible.

The Sunrider herbs were still costing me $500 a month. I was going farther into debt to continue to take the herbs. I really had no choice as I saw it. I was not about to stop any of the supplements. However, I was given the opportunity at the health food store to learn and purchase perhaps a cheaper alternative than the multi-level marketing product. To this day, I believe in Sunrider herbs, but I feel I have healed and balanced enough to limit my consumption of them. I continue to drink Sunriders' *"calli"* beverage at times. I feel this beverage has a positive effect on my overall health.

I experimented by adding and changing what I was taking. From pycnogenol to B12 lozenges, I tried to find cheaper combinations that would keep me healthy. The Juice Bar at the store had a nice commercial juicer. I was washing 50 lbs. of carrots every couple of days for the Juice Bar. I drank the fresh squeezed juices at work.

I found I was good in the store because I really cared about people and their health as I did my own. My condition had driven me right into an opportunity to become involved in helping other people heal. Eventually word of mouth got out that I had MS. People would come in the store and ask for me. Even a doctor or two sent people in to talk with me about my experiences with MS. I talked with fellow MS patients to help take the fright out of their "diagnosis" of MS. I found myself sharing my experiences with many people. I certainly suggested books to read that had helped me along the way. The thirty hours per week I worked at the store was tiring but very rewarding for my psyche. I met many people who were dealing with different and serious diseases. I realized the reading I had been doing over the last five years was paying off. My voice in the health food store environment hopefully helped others with their own health challenges.

I worked in the store for almost three years. This gave me a lot of confidence in vitamins, herbs, and the books I had surrounded myself with.

The two drawbacks from working in the store were very apparent. I was overly tired and was exposed to viruses by dealing with the public on a daily basis. This would generate uncomfortable symptoms. To combat these adversities, I would meditate before dinner, take a twenty minute walk for digestion – rain or shine – and then watch television. I would be in bed by 10:00p.m. Exhausted. Working in the store was a full day on my feet. Rewarding but tough. I remember having to hold onto the shelves of vitamins by the end of the shift. This was to help with my end of the day balance problem brought on by fatigue.

By then I was 47 years old and had been dealing with MS for six plus years. The second situation was the added exposure to viruses. Lots of people came into the health food store searching for a product to prevent or deal with a cold or flu or other health issues. On average, I caught two colds each winter season. People with MS are known to have compromised immune systems. To this day, I hold my breath to avoid anyone that looks like they may be infectious. Washing my hands with regularity has become the norm. These two drawbacks did not sway me from enjoying the experience, the people, and the knowledge I gained.

My health had stabilized over the last seven years. All the meditation, all the wheatgrass, all the sesame oil massages, all the vitamins and herbs had paid off. I felt strong enough to begin accepting new challenges. Being a "type A" personality of which I am blessed with is often part and parcel to decision making. People with MS often times fall into the "type A" personality. Upbeat positive achievers. This is not a rule, it is just an observation. I am certainly included in this group. Match my personality with a "can do" attitude and I will follow through. Attached to this "I can do" attitude is the work ethic that is required for any new demanding endeavor. As I regained my strength, I began to expand my horizons. I needed a challenge to keep me going. I discussed this with my wife Kim, and together we conceived an idea to relocate back to Hawaii where the weather was more healing, and make use of my retail experience by opening a new business.

Rather than investing a lot of money in the health food industry, we decided to open an art gallery to expand Kim's art career.

There were personal questions I had to ask myself. Could I physically handle retail sales? Could I be on my feet that long? Will I be coherent enough in the afternoon to work?

This new adventure began in 1997 when Kim flew to Oahu. Kim stayed with a friend in Kailua, Oahu for ten days. I stayed home in Washington with the cats. Within a week of arriving on Oahu, Kim sent me a map of Kauai. Obviously a pointer towards Kauai instead of any other island, Kim returned home to Port Townsend to continue her artwork while I began researching a move to Kauai. In August of 1997 I flew to Kauai. I leased a retail location in a small town on the West side, which is the dry side of Kauai. I secured a business lease in the historic town of Hanapepe and flew back to the state of Washington. Kim and I rented two storage units in Port Townsend and built second levels in each of the units with help from our neighbor in Port Townsend. We proceeded to empty our house. A huge undertaking.

By then, I was well aware of my limitations and how to deal with the symptoms of MS. I would rest often, drink lots of water, eat lots of protein, meditate with regularity and stretch in the morning. We were full speed ahead. Even with MS I knew if I paced myself and paid attention, I would be all right. I was very careful going up and down stairs.

We put our house up for sale and accepted an offer the same day. This meant we also had a very finite time to be out of the house. Thirty days from acceptance of the offer! This quick sale meant we would have to find a temporary house to live in before flying to Oahu.

The animal quarantine rules required us to have our three cats, Malcolm, Sheila and Piedmont immunized and micro-chipped on the mainland. Wait sixty days, and then we would have the legal go-ahead to fly our three cats to Oahu, Hawaii. Upon arrival on Oahu, the cats would enter a thirty day quarantine for observation. This would complete their quarantine and we would be able to continue on to Kauai. This law has now been changed to three days of quarantine, provided you comply with all the rules as required. To comply with the animal quarantine rules, we rented a house near Port Townsend for the sixty days.

Besides emptying our sold house, we crated, packed and shipped two thousand pounds of art, supplies and equipment to our new business location in Hanapepe, Kauai. Fortunately, a friend from Port Townsend, Judi Witt agreed to move to Kauai a month ahead of us. Judi's move to Kauai in December made it possible to ship equipment, etc. to her at the new gallery location. Judi was responsible for opening the new gallery until Kim and I arrived.

January 1, 1998 – Kim and I arrive on Oahu. We stayed with a friend for a month while visiting our cats five days a week at the quarantine station. This was to help the cats with the adjustment and trauma of flight. Judi opened the gallery just before Christmas 1997. Crates and boxes continued to arrive at the new gallery. Judi's help was crucial at this particular time. We would get through with a little help from our friends!

My nervous system began to react as usual by emptying my bowels several times before I even left the airport in Seattle for the flight to Oahu. Kim and I did have our customary eggs and nuts for the flight to Honolulu. All through our thirty day stay on Oahu, we followed closely our normal diet regiment. The meditation techniques we had been practicing for seven years were an asset at this time. Moving to Hawaii for the second time was stressful. The opening of an Art gallery was an addition to many other demands on us – mentally, physically and financially. Without the healing I had done during the previous seven years, I would not have been able to even think of taking on this challenge. For anyone with MS who volunteers to do tasks, only to realize the actual "doing" may be too much to handle. This is where I realized seven years of healing had come into place. This healing goal was not accomplished by accident. I worked toward this goal every hour of the day for years. The combinations I have written about in this book worked for me.

To back up a few months this decision to move was based on a check list. The pros and cons of the move we put on this list. This list weighed in favor of the move. Beginning at the top of the "to move" list was the weather. The average daily temperature in Hawaii is 78 degrees Fahrenheit. For a person healing from MS, a stable weather condition from day to day makes living with MS in Hawaii easier. Not only the freedom to be outside 365 days a year, but not having to wear layers of clothes as well. Blue sky and sunshine is a rarity in the Pacific Northwest. People with MS may find the heat and high humidity very difficult to deal with. I became acclimated to the weather after my first move and knew I could handle the heat. I had come a long way in managing MS since 1990. I had learned how to live with MS. There are no magic tricks. Attitude is my ally. A good lesson from Norman Vincent Peales "*The Power of Positive Thinking*" comes to mind. Thoughts can be controlled by knowledge. When in the throes of menacing symptoms, the mind and prayer are our first allies.

January 1, 1998 – we were officially living on Kauai with our own Art Gallery. I continued paying close attention to my health. My bowels became almost regular again. We had some financial stress but overall the meditation tool really helped with balancing the emotions. I noticed vertigo not being an issue in the mornings if at all within the first week of arrival on Oahu. I was probably thrilled to be back in Hawaii after all we had been through. I knew I could enter the art business again on my own terms. Yes, I put a bed in the storage room of the gallery. Rest and meditate. Eat protein balanced meals for energy and stamina. I had not been taking Sunrider herbs with any regularity since 1995. Since my time working at the health food store I had been keeping a vitamin tray stocked and labeled. My vitamin regimen was consistent. We put growing and drinking of wheatgrass on hold for the time being.

Before moving back to Hawaii, I was at *Dr. Rienstra's* office in Port Townsend. *Dr. Rienstra* had told me that a person I knew had inquired about me. I am not sure how this inquiry came about. *John Thoreson,* who I had known and gone to school with since the 4th grade and graduated from high school with in 1968, had just been in *Dr. Rienstra's* office. John was a representative of Carlson Labs among others. *Dr. Rienstra* used *John Thoreson's* products in his clinic. *Dr. Rienstra* gave me John's phone number. I did not wait long to call John and touch bases with him. We caught up as best we could about the last eighteen years since we had seen each other. *Dr. Rienstra* had told John of my dealing with MS. John invited me to his house in Bellevue. From that re-introduction to the present, I have leaned towards Johns' knowledge of health and healing. John gave me some new ideas about supplements I should investigate and perhaps add to my vitamin tray. One of the first products John talked about was T.E. Neesby's *"Seriphos"*. I have been taking this product for my brain and central nervous system since John told me about the product in 1997. Next was *Acidpholis* for balancing my intestinal flora to help assimilate nutrients. I had taken acidophilus but not on a regular basis. Another positive addition to my vitamin kit is *Fish Oil.* I started remembering my dreams immediately. Literally from the first time I took fish oil I found a positive difference in my sleep – deep sleep. This has to be good for my brain - maybe helping in the neuro-transmission around the MS scars I have in my brain?

John is also a representative for an Ayurvedic herb company called Ayush Herbs from Bellevue, Washington. They have an immune system enhancer called Amlaplex. A jam like concoction full of antioxidants, I have used off and on for several years. This formula was added to the vitamin and herb list as a regular requirement. John also talked about the importance of *COQ10*. To this day, I feel John Thoreson provided me with knowledge that definitely strengthens my health regimen in dealing with MS. John is also champion of the benefits of *Vitamin C* and its positive effects on the immune system.

Back to Kauai and settling on the West side. This brought a variety of positive effects and at the same time immediately presented new stress related challenges. Kim and I relied on our previous experience in starting a new business. Our good friend Judi Witt had done a great job in opening the gallery before we arrived from Oahu to Kauai. As it turned out, even the small house connected to the gallery building became available for us to rent. A 600 square foot house connected to the building that became Kim Starr Gallery. Once cleaned, Kim painted the interior while I caught a cold and became too compromised to be of any help. Fortunately, Judi was there to open the gallery daily. Even making sales while the gallery looked like a shipping and receiving room. I have to say this is a boost to anyone who opens a business - to begin making sales in the first week of operation!

Once on my feet, we built a sleeping "shelf" in the storage room for a futon and I was set. The great thing about the Hawaiian Islands is the moderate climate. We would open the door in the front of the gallery all day. I could be in my storage room lying down on "the shelf". The rickety old floor would always let me know if someone entered the gallery. We had a sink and toilet also in the storage room. With the help of *John Thoreson* I had also discovered the attributes of Kipper snacks. Canned herring was quick protein that I liked. I had a constant supply of kipper snacks and boiled eggs in my storage room. The ability to actually lay down on the job and rest was a necessity. I added a juicer to our storage unit for fresh squeezed carrot, ginger and apple juice and a refrigerator. I was staying healthy. The daily 80 degree temperature did affect my gait and added fatigue to every afternoon.

Writing this account of life with MS does not give Kim enough credit or attention. Kim never at anytime gave me reason to think she would leave me because of my battles with MS. In fact, Kim and I never wanted to have children. That was never a problem; however, I did have a vasectomy. I look at this decision as being a very sound one. As far as I can tell, having a child while dealing with MS would make life that much more difficult. I know couples do have children and maintain their marriages. My congratulations go out to them. There are definitely times that I would be unable to meet the responsibilities required of a parent. Fatigue, vertigo, and wide gait to name a few symptoms that are impossible to ignore. Having a child would be tough work when in the throes of MS symptoms. Kim and I do have six cats and believe me, this is enough responsibility!

From January of 1998 to November of 2002 we lived and worked at our gallery in Hanapepe. A walking bridge spanning the Hanapepe River was constructed in the early 1900's so school children could cross the river to get to school and is today a tourist attraction. Sugar cane and coffee fields surround the Hanapepe valley. Quite idealic in many ways. We had created quite a comfortable situation. Kim would create artwork and Judi and I would run the gallery. Hanapepe is a sleepy little town. We would average maybe eight people a day in the gallery. So I would easily be able to lie down in the storage room anytime I needed to. The small house we lived in was attached to the gallery. I could actually be sitting at the kitchen table and see people come in the front door of the gallery. This was a dream come true, owning a business in spite of having MS. I would lie down on the storage room shelf a lot more often during the summer months. The heat and humidity in Hawaii is increased during the monsoon season, about ten degrees higher. Without a trade wind, Hanapepe was hot – in the nineties. If my balance was off and or fatigue was an issue I would just lay down.

A great asset of the Hanapepe valley is the weekly farmers market. We would stock up on fresh vegetables every week. We also had a favorite fruit stand for papaya. A dozen of the best papaya for five dollars. If you have a farmers market or fruit stands in your area, I would recommend you take advantage of what they have to offer.

Almost immediately I volunteered to be part of the maintenance team to beautify both entry ways to the town. Every Tuesday another gallery owner and I would show up to mow the lawn, trim the bougainvillea and do an overall cleaning and presentation for the town of Hanapepe. We would also affix "Art night" banners on each of the two entry ways to the town announcing an art walk every Friday night. This free advertisement became a huge success for the town and our art gallery. For the next five years Kim and I put a great deal of effort into business and health. I became vice-president of a non-profit community based organization called "Hanapepe Economic Alliance". This really boiled down to being a volunteer to just do more volunteering.

The picturesque town began to shine as our efforts were rewarded by starting a trend involving many business owners as well as county participation. Hanapepe began to show this effort in subtle ways. The junk cars were hauled away. The garbage was removed from the trails, etc.

Kim and I had also acquired our own route to feed and care for a bunch of feral (wild) cats. During years we lived in the valley we caught and delivered to the Kauai Humane Society twenty seven cats for spaying and neutering. We would then take the cats back to where we caught them. We continued to care for the group and hopefully did our part in eliminating more feral cats. Every night we would walk up the hill towards the local grade school and feed fresh chicken to the feral cats. We would also take cats to the veterinarian if needed. During this time our own fenced yard held three more cats. This added up to six cats in our immediate family.

Kim and I would go to "Salt Pond Park" just a mile from home for a swim every week. An absolute beautiful location for a safe swim. Turtles and all sorts of other marine life enjoyed the safe swim of Salt Pond Park. A rock jetty a hundred yards off shore broke the surf. This provided a perfect safe location to swim for someone like myself who enjoys swimming but also is very aware of my potential fatigue and abilities while swimming. This meant Hanapepe State Park was perfect for swimming just about every day of the year. Kim and I would often go for a swim and meditate in the morning before opening the gallery. If you have access to a beach or pool you should take the time to use it. I kept the exertion on my part to a minimum. I was very careful and avoided over doing it. This shows how I had learned to be aware of my abilities as the afternoon rolls around.

Kim and I both took trips back to Washington State during those years. My health held steady. Again, the combination of meditation, diet, herbs and moderate exercise were proving to be the best way to live for me. I avoided uncomfortable symptoms as much as possible. Maintaining a rhythm for my mind and body works best.

This Hawaii lifestyle agreed with me in keeping a healthy balance. I had one trip to a neurologist during those five years and only noted on the exam I seemed to quiver at my extremities, and my wide gait was affecting my balance. But I was used to living with these symptoms. Accepting symptoms and masking them to the public and friends is normal to me. I accept these daily symptoms and do not wrap my thoughts and life around them.

There were some undeniable problems with the island lifestyle. Being so far away from family and friends was difficult. We also did not own the property in Hanapepe. In 2001 the property was offered for sale. We were not in a position to purchase the property at the asking price. The property was sold to an artist and her husband from California. We were given six weeks to move! After five years of living in the 600 sq. ft. house attached to the 1200 sq. ft. building that housed the art gallery and storage, we had to find another location to move to. Try telling a potential landlord you have six cats. We found the properties in this "cat friendly" rental pool were non-existent at the time.

Not willing to give up our family or even lighten the "herd of six" we decided to look for a rental on the island of Maui. After all, we had lived on the Big Island and Kauai why not give Maui a try? We had visited Maui before. Maui is also not a large island. If you do not take the road to Hana with its fifty-six one lane bridges or decide to drive up for a view of Haleakala Crater, you can drive around the rest of the Island easily in a day. We wanted to find a house rental near Kihei, Maui where we would open a new art gallery.

We immediately closed the doors of the Gallery in Hanapepe and began emptying the walls of art. The first week of constant packing found Kim and me on "automatic pilot". Fortunately my health was stable and besides requiring regular breaks and drinking lots of water, I remained strong. Tired, yes but we did not have the luxury of worrying about the future. We had to move it. If Multiple Sclerosis was an issue I literally do not remember even thinking about it. This is where my years of discipline in taking care of my health paid off. In this abrupt situation facing us, I was able to count on my health.

We flew to Maui and rented a 900 sq. ft. concrete block "bunker" on six acres in upcountry Kula. This rental was the only one we could find that would allow us to keep our six cats. After securing a rental, we flew back to Kauai. This brought our time to vacate Kauai down to thirty days. A much more comfortable task now that we had a place to move. Kim and I work extremely well together. We knew each other's dedication to the job at hand although we looked at this move as a positive one.

Maui has always been the number one island for art sales in the Hawaiian Islands. We moved with this added inspiration. Kim packed all the household and studio equipment. I concentrated on the art gallery. Together we were helping each other constantly. It is interesting to note in our move to Kauai we sent 2000 pounds of art and equipment. Five years later we filled a 24 foot ocean container with 30,000 pounds of gallery and household items in our move to Maui. We paced ourselves and continued to pay attention to our health. Meditation really helps with the stress of moving. Again, all the time and effort I had spent since 1990 to heal and live with MS was paying off. Moving is always stressful, but I was holding up well. We had the 24 foot container dropped in front of the Art gallery in Hanapepe. We built a ramp to roll the hand truck from the street up the 4 foot height of the container. We finished loading the steel box in three days.

The final night of Kauai found Kim, myself and our six cats almost sleepless awaiting the flight to Maui. These last forty-five days on Kauai were intense. By now we were running pretty much on automatic pilot, and when one travels with cats there has to be lots of preparation. Especially the way we go about it. We caught a ride to the airport. We landed on Maui a week before Thanksgiving. We rented a car and proceeded to move to Kula, Maui. The container was scheduled to arrive in one week. Our car would arrive from Kauai in a week. We immediately began building a temporary fence around the yard. It has always been our policy to fence our cats in. Not an easy task but necessary.

My health was holding up wonderfully. I made a note of the fatigue and some stress. I realized this would be impossible to avoid considering the circumstances. Fortunately, Maui has several good health food stores. Kim and I frequented one every day for the first week. "Healthy take out" was available so we indulged. This is not something we were used to but we were happy to have had the option.

We had to work on the rental we called the "bunker" before it was actually very livable. We slept on the concrete floor on a drop cloth for a week waiting for the container from Kauai to arrive. Kim and I also began looking for a new location for an art gallery. There were a couple of nice locations available. After settling on one, we began negotiating with the shopping center management. The process of remodeling, installing lights and preparing promotional advertising was now our main focus. We worked well beyond the 3:00 p.m. fatigue; however, all systems were running balanced.

The property we were living on in Kula was not for sale, but within sixty days of moving in, we were notified by our landlord the property would be shown, and if someone would offer him a million dollars he would sell. He had purchased the property for $425,000. This added once again to the mental unsettling, but we continued with our new gallery plans. In the fourth month of living in Kula the "bunker" was sold. This meant we were again cast into the questionable future of where to live. My health continued to be stable. However, in my overzealous way I had pulled a set of muscles in my left leg. I had done this by doing yoga sun salute exercises. Our Maui "bunker" landlord felt bad he was going to make us move, so he looked for another house for us to rent. This is not an easy task for anyone. We appreciated the effort on his part. Soon our landlord put us in touch with a man who had a rental coming available in Makawao, just eight miles from Kula. The rental house was being worked on. Not perfect for the cats, but available for us on June 1st. We had little choice with circumstances the way they were . We said we would take it. This meant we would be moving within thirty to sixty days.

At least we would not be homeless with six cats – an uncomfortable feeling for anyone. By the middle of May my sciatic nerve in my left leg was very tender. I did have a chiropractic appointment that seemed to help. I just needed to keep the upper leg iced and pay attention. With all the tentative moving and lease negotiations, Kim and I were not in a position to sign the retail lease agreement for a new art gallery. We decided to wait until we got moved to Makawao. June rolled around. We had to be out of the "bunker" rental by June 10. On this day our potential new landlord's girlfriend called us to let us know that they could not rent the house in Makawao to someone with six cats. We were taken aback by this news. We had no place to move. We were angry at this turn of events. We felt this new landlord broke his word. Especially since we were counting on this rental for six weeks. We had made no effort to locate an alternate house somewhere else because we were assured this house in Makawao.

Now this abrupt news had changed our whole program for the very near future. Kim had actually begun working on a new oil painting. Now we needed to scramble for a place to live. When I got off the phone with the news, I broke down. Kim was painting in the living room. She came into the bedroom and held on to me. I was shaking with emotion. I had not been in this position in a long time. Once I settled down and stopped the tears, I began to put a plan in motion.

Plan "B" had been on the back burner over the last seven months or since we moved from Kauai to Maui. My Mom and Dad were selling their house in Washington State and moving closer to my sisters. My sisters expressed a great desire for Kim and me to consider moving back to the mainland to be close to Mom and Dad as well. Kim and I looked one more time at the Maui News for a rental. We decided to make the move back to Washington. Yes, we had ten days to move. This meant packing another 24 foot ocean shipping container. Load and leave so to speak. I grabbed the phone and called the airlines, Matson shipping, friends in Washington and friends in Hawaii. The move seemed almost impossible at that moment but I can say that "automatic pilot" took over again. After all, Kim and I knew how to pack a container blindfolded! We had just done this seven months earlier. I was still icing the back of my left leg several times a day and sleep had improved.

Besides this non-related to MS health problem I was doing well physically. Again, the meditation we had been practicing for many years was paying off. This time crunch to pack and move in ten days gave us no time to ponder another plan. When looking in the paper for a rental you find abbreviations like NS/NP. Which means no smoking and no pets. We don't smoke but are guilty with pets. Monday rolled around and Kim was painting on the canvas she had begun a couple of days earlier. I began the morning by making thirty phone calls putting the move into place.

First was to arrange a 24 foot Matson container to be delivered to the door in Kula. This took a few phone calls. Then on to the airline reservations. A few more phone calls. Hawaiian Airlines has a policy to follow that only allows a certain amount of containers with animals on each flight. This immediately changed our departure plans. We could not leave before June11. This would be the best we could do. I made the arrangements. With these rules, we would put two cats in each of three cat containers. Hawaiian Airlines confirmed reservations for the three containers on our flight leaving Wednesday, June 11 bound for Seattle. We were that much closer.

While living in the "bunker" we had used two rooms just for storage. The container arrived and we assembled the wood ramp and began to reload the Matson shipping container bound for Seattle. We also experienced our first rain in two weeks – what timing. Then, after that first long day of packing, Kim and I wanted to reward ourselves with a nice warm shower and perhaps dinner and a little television before we packed the TV. Well, this was not to be. The hot water heater in the bunker suddenly quit working. Great. I called the landlord on his cell phone. He happened to be vacationing in California. He told me to contact a friend of his to have a look at the water heater. In the meantime, we could go to his house a few miles away and take a shower and a swim in his swimming pool. His maid would let us in. We didn't really feel like relaxing since we now had only six days left to move. On Sunday, June 8, we finished packing the container. We took the ramp apart, closed up the container and called the shipping company to pick it up.

Wednesday, June 11 arrives. Kim and I had spent the night on the floor on a futon. On the way to Kahului airport we mailed two boxes of bedding to a friend on the mainland. We then headed for the Matson office to drop off our car for shipping. We took a cab to the airport. We arrived with two bags and three containers with six cats. At the curb check-in an attendant for Hawaiian Airlines asked for our health certificates for the cats. I had no idea what she was talking about. There was no quarantine going from Hawaii to the mainland that we were aware of. But they insisted on the health certificates we did not have and knew nothing about. I called our veterinarian. Three phone calls later we hired a "mobile veterinarian" to come to the airport and examine our cats. $290 later and not so much as any cat removed from a container we had the slips of paper required. We presented this to the Hawaiian Airlines agent. Now, she said she could not let us have two cats in one container! I had talked with Hawaiian Airlines at least three times concerning this flight. We were in compliance! We have confirmations! We were told the policy just changed. However, if we could come up with a container for each of the 6 cats – in other words find three more containers – they would let us all get on the plane. I flagged down a taxicab! Took the five mile ride to the mall, purchased three more containers while the cab waited. Kim and I separated the cats and continued to try boarding. We are in compliance again! We were following the brand new rules! Now can we get on this plane to Seattle? Okay!

Fortunately, Kim and I had lived in Hawaii for fifteen years. We were aware of the potential hang-ups. This is why we had arrived at the airport five hours early. We had enough time to implement all the new demands by the airline. In fact, our Hawaiian Airline flight was also an hour late. We made our way to the gate. We sat with our fingers crossed. Every time the loudspeaker was turned on, I could feel my heart jump. Yikes. Kim and I had made it this far. An incredible demanding adventure. We followed the new rules and took two containers in the plane with us. "Candy" in one container under Kim's seat and "Elliot" under my seat. They were perfectly silent, as if they knew they had better just melt into the present circumstances and act invisible. We had a smooth flight to Seattle. I have to say that first cup of Lion coffee on the plane at 4:00 p.m. sure tasted great! Multiple Sclerosis – me? Denial. Just ignore "the MS beast." After pulling a sleepless night in Kula, and the debacles at the Kahului airport and the little things like one of the cats deciding to hide in the rafters at the Kula "bunker" just before heading out to the airport was nothing! We were on our way!

We arrived in Seattle shortly after midnight. I had arranged to pick up a rental car at the airport. Dollar Rent a Car had "upgraded" us to a Ford Mustang convertible but we now had six cat containers and two bags. This will not fit in a Ford Mustang. Fortunately, they had a Chevy Blazer to rent instead – whew. We were going to stay with a friend in Port Angeles, Washington near the Canadian and Washington border. We headed out in the Chevy Blazer. We arrived in Port Angeles at 4:00 a.m. This was also Kim's birthday! Happy Birthday Kim! We rested as best we could and tried to unwind. We spent the next seven nights in an 8x8 room with a bed. Kim and I, Malcolm, Sheila, Piedmont, Candy, Elliot and Sprout – wow – but we were all safe.

We spent the next few days building a temporary fence surrounding a thirty-five foot mobile home (our temporary dwelling), so the cats could be outside.

A beautiful new summer ahead of us – we were settling in. Kim was beautiful and glowing on her 47th birthday.

Within a week of arrival, Kim and I began our search for a new place to live. We were hoping to purchase a home. We began looking in Port Angeles. My health was holding marvelously, Kim was very supportive in all of this. She made sure I had boiled eggs, rest and meditation. Once the temporary fence was complete all of us spent a great deal of time outside. An added feature was all the wild rabbits surrounding the yard. Kim and I walked all over the streets of Port Angeles.

Now being back on the mainland, I was able to help Mom and Dad in any way I could. They had their house of thirty years under contract to sell. This was one of the steps they needed to complete before moving closer to my two sisters in Vancouver, Washington.

Port Angeles was a 120 mile trip one way to their house, plus another 140 miles to Vancouver, but I gladly helped in any way I could. If nothing else, for moral support. Moving is real tough – for anyone.

Within the first thirty days of our arrival we visited Snoqualmie. The town I grew up in. Realizing Kim and I had no idea where to look for a house, we kept our eyes open no matter where we were. Snoqualmie, Washington is a small town thirty miles east of downtown Seattle. I still have a friend that lives just six miles from where he and I were neighbors as children. We were visiting him one day and looked at houses while in the area. Snoqualmie is very rural and within thirty-five miles of SeaTac airport. Beyond being another gorgeous July day, Kim and I found ourselves attracted to a house. An obvious "fixer" built in the 1930's, we were very interested. I would often walk by this house as a child going to grade school. The school is just two blocks away. Kim and I called the real estate agent and made arrangements to view the house the following Monday. We left for the 108 mile trip back to Port Angeles for the Weekend.

Monday, July 14, Kim and I made our appointment in Snoqualmie to view the house. Within thirty minutes of walking onto the property, we decided to purchase it. Once the earnest money was accepted, we headed back to Port Angeles and our six fenced cats. On the ferry boat ride, we received a call on our cell phone – our offer was accepted. Yippee! Kim and I were overjoyed for more reasons than just the summer weather .It had only taken thirty-two days upon arrival to have an accepted offer on a house we were thrilled with.

The ride back to Port Angeles was sweet. On the health side of things I had held up well. My sciatic nerve in my leg had calmed down to normal. Now the purchase of a house was dropping my stress level by measured increments. To compare when we landed just 32 days ago we were on a roll. The thirty-five foot 1950's trailer with no running water or electricity where we were living was much appreciated. But we were looking at our first winter in six years and realizing we could not make it through the winter very comfortably in the trailer in Port Angeles. Now we had succeeded in the plan. Beyond jumping through a few of the necessary hoops to purchase a house, we were set to close escrow on Friday, August 22. The closing went like clockwork. We drove back to Port Angeles that night. On Saturday we cleaned the trailer and packed the car to the hilt. Sunday morning we loaded the cats in containers and off we went! Arriving at 1:30 p.m. at our new house we were beside ourselves with joy. We had dinner at the Puget Consumers Co-op – a large whole foods store in Issaquah. From now on we would take the days one at a time. We would not have to be in a hurry for anything. We could have the luxury of planning a strategy for just about any decision in the future. We were finally home.

I have been very fortunate with my health since our recent move. A synapse of my diaries in the back of this book will give you more of a taste of the reality of it all. Moving is a stressful situation for people and pets. Kim and I have been living in Snoqualmie a year now. Our first winter in six years ended up being a real exciting challenge for us weather wise. The worst wind in the Snoqualmie Valley in 100 years and we were here for it! My health has been consistent. Our neighbors across the street, Lori and Steve lost a tree in the windstorm in the first week of December. Steve volunteered "free firewood" if I wanted to haul it over to our house. I grabbed a wheel barrow and proceeded to help myself to the heavy rounds of fresh cut fir. Oops. Besides the pouring down rain, the wind was still blowing. I decided to work fast. Well, work fast and work stupid? I became "superman" for about thirty minutes. Two weeks later my left shoulder (I am left handed) was in pain. I could not raise my arm higher than my middle chest. What's this? Will it go away? I asked Kim and other friends. They all had shared similar experiences throughout the years. Armchair diagnosis? It will go away. Within the first month I could not lay on my left shoulder – too painful. I reached for a cat once and experienced a quick lesson of induced agony. I put up with the increasing pain until March 5. By then I was not sleeping very well and my shoulder was not improving. I made an appointment with a chiropractor. I had been hoping the situation was going to improve on its own. By the time three months had passed with no improvement, I had reached my limit with "wait and see". The chiropractor had a look and I had not broken my arm. This was a good call. He sent me to a physical therapist. Good call! The therapist diagnosed my problem as a "frozen shoulder". Whew! It has a name! For the next three months I visited the physical therapist. I also added some daily stretches and ice packs at home. The pain subsided after two months as it began to unfreeze.

Besides the work on our new home and property, Kim continues to create oil paintings for galleries that represent her work. We have taken a few trips to Vancouver, Washington to visit our families.

My health continues to be balanced. In writing this book and re-discovering the writings in my journals, I can clearly see the pattern of healing. From day to day, writings of symptoms in the "early years" to the present day journal writings with no mention of symptoms. The awareness of not being compelled to write every day is significant. As my journals point out, healing was very gradual in the beginning. It took years to get this far. The years I have been living with the diagnosis have given me a lot of practice. I practice every day. At this moment I am a little wobbly. So what? After dinner, Kim and I will go for a walk. My gait will be wide. After the evening walk I will not feel like doing anything. At 10:00 p.m. I will want to go to bed. The last paragraph is my normal life. Wow, I said it!! Normal – as I see it.

All the best.

Patrick

My Mount Rushmore

This is my mentor mountain. Each one of these individuals has their place for a reason. I am affixing my heroes' profiles on this mountain. I look to every one of these individuals to this day.

- Kim Onette Starr
- G. Gordon McIntire
- Katherine McIntire
- Jerrie and Jon Poizer
- Maryann Blessinger
- Gary Daubert
- Danny Spearman
- Thom Abbott
- Teresa Scharf
- John Dee Lucas
- Frank Branham
- Maresa and Barry Molinar
- Carole and Marty Kahn

- Jo Anne and Chuck Bullen
- Charlie Boulay
- Catharine and Frank Kuntz
- Jeff Dion
- John Pageler
- Dr. Douwe Rienstra
- John Thoreson
- Dinah Kunitake
- Annette Shortridge
- L.W. Shortridge, PhD
- Bill Abell
- Duane Leisle
- Astoria Camille
- Cliff Collins

I have a lot of friends to be thankful for everyday. This is by no means a finished list. I will add to this list, I am sure.

Chapter

12

The Future

There are no crystal balls to reveal what the future holds for a cure to Multiple Sclerosis. I am sure there will be progress. I only hope it is not confined to curing only the symptoms. I am convinced that if you follow the guidelines in this book and in those books referred to in the text, your quality of life will sustain you into the future and reveal new medical procedures and non-invasive drugs that will hopefully cure MS.

You now hold a gift, a gift that has been given with hope.

Hope that you will grasp this raft of life as it floats in a sea of despair and embrace a happier, healthier life in the future.

L.W. Shortridge, PhD

Chapter

Interesting One Liners

- *Never give up on yourself*

- *Placebo shows us the power of the mind*

- *Readers Digest has it right – laughter is the best medicine*

- *You are what you think*

- *You are what you eat*

- *Don't dilly-dally*

- *Dairy digestion is difficult*

- *John Thoreson is a genius*

- *Prayer is free (no matter which God you praise)*

- *You can lead a horse to water but you can't make him drink*

Diary Timeline Synapse

The following synapse of seven volumes of diaries are just that. A synapse. I entered this snapshot version in this book to point out the simplicity and the importance of keeping a daily log. There are days the diary became long winded and very heartfelt in emotion and malaise. Other days, the diary was a mere calendar of the day with no entries. A diary is a healing tool. Begin now.

July 6, 1989 Diary begins

September 3, 1990 - I am experiencing yucky symptoms. Woke up with no sight, just strobes and fell to the bedroom floor.

September 5 - I have an appt. with *Dr. Rienstra*. Diagnosis. More likely an inner ear infection

September 6 - Feel bad. Very dizzy all day long

September 10 - Went to a different doctor. Had blood drawn

September 12 - No problem with blood. Awoke at five in the morning with diarrhea, anxiety and shortness of breath

September 19 - I buy book on Transcendental Meditation, add aerobic exercise, weights

September 21 – I don't feel very good

September 25 – Panic to tears uncontrollable, dizzy always

October 11 – 11:00 a.m. Neurologist exam ordered. Magnetic Resonance imaging scan – Bremerton

October 12 – Results from MRI scan – Multiple Sclerosis

October 18 – I see *Dr. Linda Showler ND*. Try a homeopathic approach. Not good for me. I also recommend Kim to see *Dr. Showler*

October 27 – Instruction for a class on Transcendental Meditation

October 30 – Our last evening of TM practice

November 3 – We receive our TM mantras

December 23 – I am chronic with MS symptoms. I feel sorry for Kim. My depression brings me to tears.

January 21, 1991 – We begin floor sanding in our Port Townsend house

January 31 – My right hand twitches – worries me

February 1 – Hand quits twitching

February 2 – Go to Seattle. Lunch at Sunlight. Seems the "on the go" makes my bowels active. Went three times in Seattle. Tired

February 4 – Night bowel problems

February 6 – Kim begins 50"X60" boat painting

February 7 – Oatmeal for dinner. Many times to the bathroom

February 8 – Have papaya juice at 4:00 p.m. Will not have dinner – feel full

February 9 – Lunch was Basmati rice, celery and sunflower seeds. I also had a piece of butter and bread

February 13 – Our wedding anniversary. Fountain Café for lunch. I have a bowl of clam chowder

February 14 – I must learn to not be in a hurry. I must calm down and make this a point. It seems the old eat and run habits sneak in at certain meals. I then throw my Vata off so I become nervous. Tonight I am nervous for business reasons – all self induced

February 15 – Have appointment with *Dr. Rienstra*. Ativan prescription ran out. My weight is 118 with clothes and boots on

February 16 – Kim finishes 50"X60" boat painting. Took a nap as usual

February 17 – At the gallery in Port Townsend. Take a nap in the car. We are eating Maharishi vitality mix. I ate soaked raisons at 2:30 p.m. – really made my bowels move. It seems like I feel sick before bowel movements – then fine thirty minutes afterwards

February 22 – Kim and I go to gallery. I take a nap in the car at 3:00 p.m. – a little light headed though

February 24 – I feel a little spacey but have a good day. It is 7:45 p.m. I am tired. Kim and I talk about the art business. This winds me up but I can handle this much better because I am practicing TM

February 26 – Went to Bellevue to pick up posters, (cats) I feel weak but better than most trips. No sleeping pill. Slept off and on all night

February 27 – Slept 1.5 hours then awakened frightened/ did not feel good. Took ½ of an Ativan. Slept until 6:30 a.m.

March 1 – I started my sesame oil massage. I feel it really helped! This could be my best day in months! I really feel this massage had a direct influence on my physiology

March 2 – Stayed at gallery from 10:20 a.m. to 8:30 p.m. Gallery walk. I am tired a few times. Too busy for nap. Go to bed at 10:00 p.m. ½ sleeping pill. Also: Saturday morning was my second day of massage

March 3 – Awakened at 5:30 a.m. Slept well. Took ½ Ativan. Third morning of massage. Weight lifting. Did feel a little dizzy in evening. Bowel movement at 9:00 p.m. probably because of late dinner. 6:45. I was tired when we arrived home. I took a nap till 6:00 p.m. Then had a ten minute meditation. I have been eating cooked apples with raisins for lunch and dinner – it seems to work well for me

March 4 – fourth massage. Pruned trees. In the afternoon I cried for a while – Kim comforted me. I felt so helpless. Took ½ Ativan sleeping pill

March 5 – fifth massage. I do much better today. Still have some dizziness and bowel problems

March 6 – Potluck at *Dr. Rienstras*. Group meditation. Somewhat dizzy but I probably needed a nap

March 7 – One of my best days ever

March 8 – I feel I am much better after eight days of massage – symptoms much less. I am working on taxes – this does stress me out

March 10 – I am weak. Took nap in car. Ten days of massage though. I ate bread with almond butter & blackberry jam at lunch – ½ piece. This is real different for me in the last five months. Have three bowel movements – one at 8:30 p.m. It seems my bowel movements are delayed because of massage.

March 14 – We head for Oregon. Arrive in Roseburg on the 15th. Look around the town, feel real good

March 18 – Spend the last couple of days looking at land

March 19 – Leave for Port Townsend. I have gotten tired of driving a couple of times but this is my own fault. The one "cheese" on vegetables meal in Roseburg was definitely a warning to quit dairy. We do not do very well keeping up with our Ayurvedic diet on the road. After five days we are ready to head home.

March 20 – Great to be home. I am weak. Breakfast at Salal. I have white pancakes for breakfast – pretty spacey after this. I have my first sesame oil massage in five days – I really needed to come home to my routine

March 21 – Kim and I start hanging French doors. I do not take a sleeping pill

March 22 – I receive a call from Dinah Kunitake from Holualoa, Hawaii. We talked about Chinese herbs. Second day in a row after trip for sesame oil massage. I did do dry massage during trip though. I feel a little spacey and weak. I have three bowel movements before 11:30 a.m. about noon I cried uncontrollably. I think I made a mistake and took the flax oil and cottage cheese about forth-five minutes before lunch. I did the same thing a couple of months ago and had a tough afternoon emotionally.

March 28 – We go to Seattle to deliver posters. I have cream of asparagus soup and sweet potato pie

May 19 – My parent's forty-sixth wedding anniversary. I figure out small meals are best for me

May 21 – I am dizzy. I feel I am eating too much sugar

May 30 – I cried today.

June 8 – JoAnne works first day!!

June 19 – I take first amount of *Sunrider* herbs. Feeling good after *Sunrider*.

June 21 – I cut out all sugar

June 23 – I feel good – lightheaded off and on. I sell pastel to client at the gallery

June 24 – I am light headed

June 26 – I feel good but a little wavy. Gary Daubert leaves. We had a good time. Gary begins taking *Sunrider*. I take *Sunrider* three times. We play catch.

June 27 – I feel good but a little wavy

June 28 – I feel good but still dealing with equilibrium. Kay Harper comes by – I finally get to meet her. Kay has been in a wheel chair with MS for ten years. She has helped me through some very tough emotional times over many phone calls

July 1 – Kim buys book on healing as a child

July 2 – I feel great with *Sunrider*

July 19 – I played twenty minutes of tennis today. Also fourth day of weight lifting. My 30th day of *Sunrider*. For the first month, I have overall been much improved. Some floating still

August 2 – Obviously I have not written in my diary for some time. I feel so much better on the whole. A bit of float/spacey while walking. Emptied bowels but still did not feel very good. Maybe over doing it. Somewhat sad. Kim helped comfort me.

August 4 – Sesame oil massage. Feel better – still early bowel movement – ½ dozen bowel movements throughout the day.

August 5 – I would say a perfectly healthy day. I have to remember the symptoms continue to come and go. I may feel lousy for an hour one day then great then lousy the next

August 6 – Mildly floaty but feel good anyway

August 7 – Feel good all day. Meditation at Dr. Rienstra's

August 12 – Work in gallery. Feel a little flitzy. Probably not enough exercise during the day.

August 13 – Sesame oil massage, stretch/yoga Sun salutes. Felt yucky in the early evening. Symptoms

August 14 – I begin using visualization techniques to heal. I feel yucky off and on in the afternoon, however other symptoms subside

August 15 – sesame oil massage, work, felt wonderful

August 16 – Not good sleep. Feel good. No bowel movement

August 17 – Busy in gallery – feel good

November 16 – Update. Three months have passed. Continued *Sunrider* foods. As an overview of the three months, I have many more good to perfect days. Therefore I have not been writing in the journal. The times when I feel lousy have lessened. Instead of days feeling lousy, I am now down to an afternoon or evening here and there. However, I realize the MS cloud is present. I try to ignore it as often as I can. My energy level is overall better by far. I feel *Sunrider* is the reason. Business has had its ups and downs the last three months. As far as working out, walks and daily exercise, and massage I am not keeping up as I was three months ago. Therefore I feel this is an indication I feel much better. I feel I control a lot of how I feel. I overdue my work load at times.

November 19 – We leave to proof a poster printing of "Moonshine in the Snow" and "Snow Scene" in Seattle. Astoria, our friend goes with us. Arrive home at 5:30 p.m. I feel a lot better after I eat. Weakness is present today. Dizziness is not. Call George? He has seen *Dr. Swank. Dr. Swank* says we are wasting our time, especially trying to regenerate the myelin sheath.

November 20 – Did not sleep soundly last night. However, felt good until getting weak around 2:00 p.m. Sesame oil massage and exercise though. Good mental attitude until Evening. Worked all day – probably overdid it. The evening was just okay.

November 21 – I feel excellent

November 22 – I had a really good day. Sesame oil massage.

November 23 – Feel good. Sesame oil massage. Ten pushups. Yoga sun salutes. Work at gallery but walk briskly to uptown post office. Evening I feel some symptoms – bowels. But a little off kilter. Note: I did not have flax oil. I believe this is of interest.

November 26 – Work out in a.m. – ten push up's, four sun salutes. On and off all day. I feel lousy. The "yuk" feeling followed by depression and my gait is swaying. I feel better after eating in late afternoon. In the morning I had oatmeal and soymilk. I am subjected to Kim's cold for the last five days. I am questioning my immune system.

November 27 – Thanksgiving. Sesame oil massage. Two egg whites with breakfast. Felt really positive and good. Two more egg whites at lunch. So I believe I am protein deficient. My depression was low, my energy level up. Since I did quite a bit after two hours after breakfast and lunch, my equilibrium was slight but I feel that the "yuk" feeling of the last two days is gone.

November 28 – Egg whites for breakfast. I feel real good. However, do have Kim's cold symptoms.

November 29 – Cold symptoms, scratchy throat, however, I feel good. The "bad" feelings are non-existent. Once again, I feel the egg whites are really making a difference. I believe I was missing something in my diet.

November 30 – I catch Kim's cold, but still feel good.

December 2 – Cold is out of head and now somewhat in my chest, but overall better. Still working on eggs and tempeh etc. for protein.

December 6 – Pick up Andrew Carpenter at airport in Seattle

December 7 – Art Show in Gallery

December 8 – I have done very well physically, however tiring, with symptoms of weak legs to follow. I feel very well the day after

December 9 – Have a good day physically. Sent out lots of Christmas cards. I have been taking Spirulina for four days. A good source of B12? I feel it is very beneficial.

December 12 – Feel good, some fatigue

December 13 – Begin evening primrose oil and mega balance multi-vitamin

December 14 – Make lentil soup for lunch. End up with a very gastrointestinal evening – bad night.

December 16 – feel very good

December 17 – Go to Seattle, lousy food at Julia's Restaurant – spicy. Had wobbly afternoon, but not that bad

December 18 – Feel good, hardly any sleeping pill last night

December 19 – Feel Great!

December 20 – Work all day – nervous system wound up; however, body handles it well. Basically I feel fine. About a week has gone since eating Mega Balance 44, Spirulina, and Evening Primrose oil, two Cod Liver oil. I feel there is a definite change in energy ability. Sesame oil massage.

December 21 – A great week. Started stretching and small weights. Vitamins, etc. good. I feel overall better with energy.

December 25 – Christmas. Sunny 50 degrees. I stacked wood, Kim baked. Had dinner at the Fountain Café with Andrew Carpenter. Wonderful Christmas with Kim, Tami and Andrew. However, stayed until 11:30 p.m. and was wasted when I arrived home. Kim could not sleep. I had a bowel problem. Certainly brought on by what and how I ate. Rough night until approximately 2:30 a.m.

December 26 – I feel really good all day. Kim and I spend most of the day at home. I really feel exercise and vitamins are key. Nuplus from Sunrider at times when I expect weakness. First in morning

December 28 – We take Andrew to Airport. Pasta at home for dinner. I end up with lots of gas, but feel good. Kim and I go to gallery until 7:40 p.m. We work on sign.

December 29 – Kim and I work in gallery. We hang all posters up over the display cases. Kim designs and we work on side sign for Bishop Hotel building. I feel good until 5:30 p.m. I was kind of yucky but only until I ate. I worked out this morning with biceps/triceps, etc. I feel good. I would say I do not have MS at times when I feel like this

December 30 – Kim and I work in gallery making plans. I feel good. Work out light in morning

December 31 – I feel good

January 1, 1992 – (Friday) Happy New Year! I do morning breathing exercises (Pranayama) taught to us by Dr. Rienstra at our TM class. Kim and I meditate twice. The wind is really blowing but not that cold out. I go for a walk before meditation

January 2 – I work out with weights

January 4 – I work out with weights, 2 new exercises – waist to shoulder lifts/bicep weights

January 5 – Great day

January 6 – I work out, I feel great. Bowels good etc. We work around house

January 7 – I get up at 7:15 a.m. – awake a little earlier. However ½ sleeping pill last night – sleep well. I make pumpkin muffins and tofu for breakfast. I feel good all day until I realize I had four bowel movements today. So, I believe I may have eaten too much protein at one time. Kim and I go to Bread and Roses Coffee House. We share an espresso; the coffee makes me feel rough. I go for an evening walk. I have a pretty darned good day symptom wise

January 8 – Took the 9:25 Kingston ferry. Deliver posters to Winn Devon Editions. Pick up paintings at Leather Furniture Company. Have lunch at the Sunlight restaurant. We head for Blaine to deliver paintings. We end up bringing all the art back. Shepherd Gallery cancels order. I feel good all day. I have a piece of vegan apple pie at the Sunlight. Also, the tofu salad. Felt good, long drive. I am happy how I held up

January 9 – We have meeting in Gig Harbor. I feel good all day. Amazing to be so busy yesterday then this trip the next day. Lousy lunch at Gig Harbor but we just don't eat much of or rely on one sandwich and carrot juice

January 10 – Feel good. Windy in Port Townsend. I talk with a man and woman who have MS

January 11 – I get up and begin to exercise, however, feel bowels are full, and so I stretch only. I feel ok. Have morning bowel movement, and then eat breakfast. Go to work at 10:00 a.m. I don't feel real sharp in afternoon. The "yuks" are upon me, but I know it will pass. I have been feeling so great. I took a Korean white ginseng at lunch – it is 6:30 p.m. and I am feeling better. Five bowel movements today. For the last hour or so I have become relaxed massaging Kim. We also went for a walk. I feel much better than at 4:00 p.m.

January 12 – I worked out in morning – feel good. Go to work at 10:30 a.m. Very slow in gallery. Nice weather, but overcast. I am kind of frail walking but I walked uptown and then back to the gallery about 3:00 p.m. I took a Valerian capsule. I come home and meditate. Kim makes a wonderful broccoli curry. I feel better after dinner. I think my equilibrium is mildly off

January 13 – Kim and I both go to gallery. Slept real good last night. Feel fine during day. Around 5:00 p.m. when Kim goes to class I feel nervous. I stay at gallery until after 6:00 p.m. I have anxiety. I believe this was controllable because I know better, so a lesson was learned. I had a sesame oil massage in the morning. This felt great. Financial stress is a problem. We have been waiting for a $6320 check that did not show up. The gallery backed out of the deal, bills are due. I make biscuits for dinner tonight for Kim to come home to. Also washed the dishes.

January 14 – I wake about 6:15 a.m. – slept good. I get up, sesame oil massage. Breakfast over by 8:20 a.m., meditate. I believe this is a good direction so I can get all my contexts done in the morning. No anxiety now. Still doing breathing exercises. 6:00 p.m. I just had a ½ bowl of corn puffs and vanilla soy milk plus 1/3 teaspoon of Sucanat as a treat. Most of the day was good. However, I am going to say at 3:00 p.m. I had an eight ounce carrot juice and wheat grass. Felt the positive effects. I believe at times I am eating too much almond butter

January 15 – I have a sesame oil massage. I work out/add exercise. Feel good. No almond butter. Change to biscuits and soy/corn puffs. Feel good. A very positive day. Also, Nuplus and carrot juice and wheatgrass. A Transcendental Meditation meeting at 7:30 p.m. Slow at Gallery. I walk up to food co-op.

January 16 – I to work. I feel good. I will have to say I am much better than a week ago.

January 17 – I lift weights, feel good. Go to work at 11:00 a.m. really symptom free except some gait variances. I meditate at work. Busy in Gallery. Since I was up at 6:15 a.m. my fatigue set in by 4:00 p.m. Some light headedness. Just tired. I go to the bathroom a few times. For dinner Kim makes curried broccoli/dairy free pumpkin pie. Excellent.

January 19 – Beautiful day. Busy in gallery. 8 oz. carrot juice/wheatgrass and felt the positive effects. Oil massage in morning.

January 20 – I work. Gorgeous day. Lift a full set of weights. Fifteen pushups. I take small amount of "KM", ½ Sunrider herb. Feel good all day. Sometimes weak at legs, but I am used to it. That is why I believe in regeneration.

January 21 – Gallery is closed. Kim and I have tea at Bread and Roses. 2nd day of "KM" the liquid supplement. Also, ½ dose of Sunrider. Feel great all day. This could be the best day I have had in six months. I must remember that

January 22 – I work out/lift full set. Best work out since beginning again. 3rd day of KM. 1 tablespoon morning and night. I feel my legs are steady and more energy overall. I feel great all day

January 23 – Sesame oil massage. I feel excellent

January 24 – I work out heavy

January 25 – Sesame oil massage. Feel good all day. Walk up to Food Co-op.

January 26 – Rough sleep but not expected. No sleeping pill for 2 ½ hours. Then took one and screwed up the balance. Good day at gallery however.

January 27 – Leave at 8:25 a.m. for Seattle. Have a waffle and blueberries at Sunlight Restaurant. No problem bowel wise. Lunch a tofu salad. Rainy day. For dinner I have Rice cereal and soy milk. Feel real good

January 28 – Nice weather but rained last night. I work out with weights this morning. We go to Bread and Roses for tea. I have a couple of sips of espresso. Feel good all day. Take a nap at 3:00 p.m. I feel mildly yucky in evening. However, feel the pistachio on an empty stomach was not a very good balance, so I do expect this is the problem. Calli tea in evening feels good. It is 8:00 p.m. all is well.

January 29 – Windy day. Some depression. Slept in until 9:00 a.m.

January 30 – Have lunch with Charlie Boulay. I am a little wavy today. However, worked out this morning.

January 31 – Work around house in kitchen. I am kind of unsteady. Kim makes cookies. I eat 3 at 4:00 p.m. Feel good at night, and then eat cereal for dinner.

February 1 – (Saturday) lousy weather. I have been taking less Sunrider for three weeks. However, had gastric problems/not a great day. Evening bowel problems. 10:00 p.m. Kim spends whole day on kitchen tear out. I feel better than Friday but realize off day

February 2 – I sleep until 9:00 p.m. have a good day physically, but lousy weather

February 3 – I work out heavy. Kim and I work in kitchen. Gorgeous day. Best of year. I feel great all day. Walk awhile. I double up on Sunrider last night. I feel this makes a difference. Bowels are fine. Have a movement at 4:15p.m.

February 6 – Gorgeous day. Sesame oil massage.

February 7 – Rough night last night. No sleeping pill. Friday evening some bowel problems

February 9 – Slow at gallery. Overcast weather. Feel good but weak since we stayed up until 1:00 a.m.

February 11 – Gorgeous day. I feel a little dizzy and depressed but actually feel good otherwise.

February 12 – Nice day. Some vertigo. Begin Ginkgo Biloba at 3:00 p.m. from *Dr. Rienstra*. ½ sleeping pill. Lifted weights in morning

February 13 – (Thursday) our tenth wedding anniversary. Breakfast at Salal Restaurant. Begin pruning trees. I feel good. Very little vertigo

February 15 – Great day physically. ½ sleeping pill

February 16 – I wear myself out, so symptoms arrive. Not enough to eat. Lack protein. Feel faint and gait is affected in evening. I eat two egg whites in evening. Feel okay but stomach is tender.

February 17 – I ate more protein and felt better. Walked long way uptown after lunch. Thirty people in gallery

February 18 – I boosted my protein intake by eating two eggs. Also, two Spirulina in morning and two at lunch. I believe I overdid it. Some constipation. So I should back off by ½ the protein. I feel this may work well. I feel good today

February 19 – Go to Seattle. Ice Skate (Kim). Deliver posters to Winn. Feel good. Ate breakfast before I left. One Spirulina. Overall, I did real well. Ice skating was easier

February 21 – I ordered wheatgrass juicer

February 23 – I work in gallery. I feel lousy when I get home. I am drained so symptoms arrive

February 24 – I lift weights

February 25 – I feel excellent. I do overlook some weakness in gait

February 26 – Early ferry to Seattle. I work out first. We ice skate. I feel excellent

February 28 – I worked out

March 1 – Sesame oil massage

March 2 – I lift two sets of weights. Feel yucky around 3:00 p.m. but feel good in evening

March 3 – Feel okay but some depression because of lack of business happenings

March 4 – Work out with heavy weights – two sets. Leave for Seattle at 8:25 a.m. I am pretty wasted all day. I strained in morning and did not recover

March 5 – No sleeping pill last night. Gastric fullness from vegetarian chili at Elliot Bay Book Store. I learned lesson. I overdid it yesterday. Symptoms all day because of it. Then no sound sleep last night. So I am not doing very well. Wobbly and tired and sensitive stomach. I will take it easy Friday.

March 6 – Work part of the day only

March 9 – I feel good. We arrange flight to Phoenix, AZ

March 12 – the last few days have been real good. Evening wobbles but controllable – otherwise feel good

March 13 – Feel real good. Kim and I go to lunch at Salal

January 22, 1993 – I have decided to add a bit on this diary. Since I haven't written in this journal consistently for ten months I will write an overview from memory. I can say life goes on with MS. A factor on a weekly basis throughout 1992. However, every week there are days when I am doing just fine. Only a few times do I remember unmanageable symptoms which are the times when symptoms such as vertigo and "yuk" stay with me for a whole evening. I have led pretty much a normal life because of my attempt to balance my symptoms. We have been growing and drinking wheatgrass for about six months. I have balanced days. I read, meditate and take my diet very seriously daily. I have not been doing oil massage every day which I feel I am missing. Not enough regular exercise. However I still have had only two real uncomfortable times I remember in the last ten months. We walk thirty minutes after dinner every night. I do use a sleeping pill most every night. I have not cried in the last ten months but have been depressed a few times a month but not for very long. I have been cutting down on herb intake to save money. But I sure know how they have helped me. I believe I am going to watch regeneration stepped up in 1993.

January 23 – Cold. Health very good.

January 24 – I feel good most of the day. 2nd day I stretched in the morning. Begin again the weights and stretching, five pushups. I feel my left eye is much worse than before the exacerbation of 1990, so I will work to strengthen it

January 25 – Awaken at 9:00 a.m. Slept well. ½ sleeping pill. Take the day off. Have tea downtown. Walk all around Port Townsend but realize hunger causes symptoms and wobbly legs. Drank wheatgrass juice at 4:00 p.m. take Sunrider herbs and stretch

January 26 – First real afternoon working on taxes. No business. Rough night sleep last night until I take ¾ of an Ativan sleeping pill around 1:30 a.m. Felt good all day. Exercised/stretch fourth day in a row. No wheatgrass today

January 30 – Nice day. I feel good. Non-dairy pizza for dinner

January 31 – Feel good health wise. ½ sleeping pill last night. Stretched in morning and pushups. Two meditations

February 12 – Beautiful day. The last two weeks my Sunrider consumption has been Quinary three times a day plus a Mega Balance multiple vitamin and Cod Liver oil. Three ounces of wheat grass juice daily. We have been growing our own wheatgrass for over a year now

February 13 – our eleventh wedding anniversary. Kim and I have dinner at the Fountain Café. No dairy and no garlic. Garlic is too harsh on my bowels

February 14 – Health fine. We walk around town. I come back and spend ten minutes on the step climber for exercise

February 18 – Kim has a cold

February 20 – Snow in the morning

February 24 – Kim and I both work. Third day of "Healing and the Mind" on TV by Bill Moyer

February 25 – Worked out again. Probably two weeks in a row now

February 26 – I feel fine. Wheatgrass in evening. Mary Kaiser and I talk about sharing their retail space

March 1 – I work out with pretty heavy weights. Trim trees. Might have overdone myself. Some vertigo occasionally

March 2 – Fourth night of wheatgrass

March 5 – Stressful day. Had a physical scare. Vertigo ant teeth chattering for ½ hour

March 6 – Feel much better. Eat slowly!

March 8 – Deliver crate to Lynden Air Freight. Felt good all day

March 10 – Begin gallery closing day

March 14 – Stressful these days with closing sale. Lifting weights and stretching regularly now

March 15 – Moved a lot of stuff to storage. Felt vertigo coming on all day and the yuks

March 16 – Increased protein. 1 full egg with the cereal. Egg and tuna fish at lunch. Evening I am feeling better. An uncomfortable twenty hours off and on

March 17 – Kim poached Cod fish. Some lessening of vertigo. Not feeling so yucky

March 18 – Poached Cod for lunch. Busy in gallery. Some vertigo lightened. Gary Daubert coming over Saturday to power wash house

March 21 – Gary falls off roof! Ambulance arrives. Gary is okay after three hours in x-ray

March 29 – Went to Seattle. Sunlight Restaurant for waffle/blueberries – bad idea? Pick up picture framing. Pasta for lunch. Honey Bear for Kim. Not enough sleep last night. Bowels flushing in evening. Tuna sandwich for dinner

March 30 – Feel fine in morning, but not much energy. Some vertigo

October 11 0 It has been six months since writing in my journal. I have gained my health balance back enough to attempt to open a new art gallery in Scottsdale, Arizona. I pay so much attention to my health, I will be fine

October 17 – Arrive at gallery at 10:00 a.m. Few people around. Leave at 3:30 p.m. I go for a swim

October 18 – Tough evening physically

October 21 – 7:00 p.m. I went home and laid down in the afternoon to be ready for Gallery walk

November 6 – I pack a big lunch with pasta. Mild vertigo before I use the bathroom

November 11 – Meditation twice a day. Keeping a positive attitude

November 25 – Thanksgiving at Roger/Diane's house. How warming for me!

November 27 – A little bit spaced out and weak, however this will pass. Two eggs for lunch and raw broccoli. Think positive

November 28 – Gorgeous day. Slept well. Egg/rice for lunch

December 2 – I have my haircut by Juno next door. I am fighting off a cold – sore throat, etc. Challenging

December 3 – Seems like my imbalance is better. Stuffy nose but not as miserable as yesterday. I really consumed the vitamin C and water

December 4 – I did not sleep at all last night. I stayed at the gallery only an hour and went home with a cold. A nasty one complete with runny nose

December 5 –I stay home to recuperate from cold

December 6 –I am at work. Feel weak but am recovering. Slept fine last night

December 12 – I worked noon to 4:00 p.m.

December 13 – I slept real well last night but have some vertigo today with bowel flushing

December 18 – Some depression is creeping in after a few days of vertigo. I quit eating bread again yesterday

December 20 – Feeling much better. Added more protein

December 21 – Now that I have lived in the Phoenix Valley I am getting an impression of the weather, smog commute, etc. Fountain Hills is better.

December 22 – Appt. with medical doctor – wants me to stop taking Ativan. He is concerned about muscle loss

December 25 – Christmas. Kim and I talk on the phone. I am so fortunate

December 27 – I feel fine. I started working tricep exercises – a good sign for me

December 28 – Rough night – bowel flushing

December 29 – I feel woozy but taking time to relax and close eyes at Gallery. I have the sensation of my hair on my head being pulled – signs of stress. Did exercises and weights, pushups, meditation and prayer.

January 17, 1994 – Monday earthquake in California – 6.6. I have taken protein powder from Shaklee distributor from gallery across street

January 19 – Gorgeous day. 4:00 p.m. I cry with anxiety and depression. I call Kim

January 20 – My middle right finger knuckle has been swollen for a week. It is hard to straighten out the finger. I have been taking Evening Primrose oil, 1000 MG/day from natures Life. The finger is so swollen it seems the skin will split. This is the first time ever

January 26 – Kim arrives a week from today – yippee!

February 2 – Kim arrives – I break down in her arms

February 4 – Arizona Irish wins the horse race.

February 13 – Our 12the wedding anniversary!

March 15 – Jeff Yeager, property manager says "Rodeo Press" will be taking over our space

March 16 – It has been two weeks since I stopped taking Ativan. I had three rough nights of no sleep. The MD prescribed Elavil. I took it a couple of times and stopped. I did not like how it made me feel. I have been taking a homeopathic and also drinking bedtime tea. I am sleeping well

March 17 – Two yoga "Sun Salutes"

March 26 – Beverly from the book store next door brings me a book "A History of the Middle East"

March 28 – Beverly from next door book store is moving out

March 29 – I lift weights in the morning

April 2 – Elavil last night. That is it – sleep fine except for some wobbly gait in my evening walk

April 17 – 100 degrees in Scottsdale. We are all but out of the gallery location

April 18 – Gorgeous – go for another swim. Move more stuff to storage in Scottsdale – all but moved. Head for Port Townsend with U-Haul

June 12 – Kim's birthday – we go to downtown Port Townsend. We have emptied the rental truck from Scottsdale. We are completely moved out of Arizona

September 1994 thru September 1995 found me working at Waterfront Naturals health food store. I read and learned a lot about supplements. I stopped taking Sunrider herbs from the multi-level marketing company which I used since 1991. I stopped because of the price of Sunrider. However, kept drinking their Calli beverage. For the last ½ of 1995, I used, on a regular basis – Pycnoginol, multi-vitamin by Nature's Life, vitamin E by Twin Lab, Enerchee by Nature's Way, B-complex by Twinlab, Spiruling, Coq10, and Ginkgo Biloba three times a day. How do I feel? Better overall in the last year and a half. My vitamin, herb regimen has made a very noticeable change in my stamina. Better than normal. Balance the same as eighteen months ago. Vision, worse than eighteen months ago

December 30 I work at health food store. Overall feel very good. I am tired at the end of the day

December 31 – I have headache but probably from lower back and work at the store

January 2, 1996 – Cloudy – took two Calms Forte and slept well last night. Reading Julian Whitacre

January 3 – Go to Seattle and deliver posters. I take two Calms Forte for sleep. I have some displeasure before sleep

January 4 – We go to Bread and Roses for coffee. Keeping up with meditation. Feel real good. Mild spot of depression over weather. We build fire today in the furnace

January 5 – I wake up okay – then I have three bowel movements in a row. Real weak. Back to bed. Upset stomach, flu symptoms. Bad, bad, bad. Now bowel control. Worst night in years – cancelled work at health food store. Literally cold sweats at times. Lots of prayers

January 6 – I feel a little better. Did not eat at all yesterday. ½ protein drink of Nature's Life Pro 96 in the morning, then back to bed. I am weak. Touch and go

January 7 – I rest all day. Protein drink, gain appetite back. Sensitive stomach

January 8 – Weak but better, feel like I am going to be fine. Give Gary Kaiser a listing for our house in Port Townsend ($89,500

January 9 – Julie Duke calls – a friend with MS needs mental support. Happy to give it

January 10 – We leave at 5:30 a.m. to fly to Sacramento, California

January 11 – What a drive from Auburn, California to Santa Rosa. Found some beautiful country, however just no improvement except weather. A real windy assention and descention to Santa Rosa – except for the gunshot last night! We are fogged in. We do not feel this area to be where we would want to live. We leave for our drive to San Francisco, on highway 101 at 11:30 a.m. Had a real good night's sleep. Stay overnight in Seaside, CA

January 14 – Had a look at Carmel Valley. Very overcast but not raining – feel very good physically

January 15 – Martin Luther King Day. We walked around Sacramento for hours. I have a cheese-less pizza for dinner but I do say I consumed more saturated fats than my normal intake. Feel fine though

January 17 – I feel fine. Kim is fighting a cold. Taking lots of vitamin C and Echinacea

January 22 – I feel fine

January 27 – Cold outside. I feel good. Amazing for the amount of stuff we have been doing

February 9 – I work eight hours at the health food store – tired

July 25 – The last five months have been full of all sorts of life experiences. Overall, a mild winter and my health was okay. Some loss of strength. I am still working at the health food store part-time

August 2 – Mom and Dad visit

August 18 – Exercise begins again

August 23 – I work out with weights

August 24 – I work all day at the health food store. Go home and rest for the evening

August 27 – Go to Mom and Dad's. Kim has baked two non-dairy berry pies

August 29 – I worked out

August 30 – I work at store. I feel kind of tired

August 31 – Long day at store – I am tired

September 3 – I work out consistently for the last few weeks

September 26 – I do not feel very good – tired. We adopt the next door neighbor's stray cat – we name him Piedmont

September 27 – We go to Silverdale – I feel like crap coming home. Fatigue

September 28 – Worked at health food store. Fatigue

October 5 –I do not sleep all night. Kinetic sculpture race in Port Townsend

November 30 – I work at health food store. Overall, my health has been good

December 5 – I work out with weights as usual. Didn't sleep very well last night though

December 6 – No sleep. The paper mill stinks all night

January 12, 1997 – Kim and I are trying to get over horrendous colds. Wow, what a bad virus. The strength of the virus was scary. It made my skin hurt for three days. Uncontrollable coughing

February 13 – Our wedding anniversary

February 26 – Kim flies to Honolulu

April 20 – I worked at health food store yesterday

April 30 – I work out with weights, four Sun Salutes. Cold and windy in Port Townsend

May 3 – I work at health food store

May 9 – I am fighting a cold virus

May 10 – I work at store. Gorgeous weather

May 14 – Hawaii Governor Cayatano sighs quarantine limit bill

June 1 – Work at health food store

June 5 – I spend day with John Thoreson

June 6 – I have ferocious headache

June 7 – Work at health food store

June 14 – Work at health food store

June 21 – Work at health food store

June 22 – Feel lousy. MS feeling yuk

June 28 – Worked at health food store

June 29 – Rest

July 4 – My last day working at health food store

July 12 – Talk with John Thoreson

July 17 – Take Gary out for coffee – his seventh year of sobriety

July 18 – Stayed at John Thoreson's last night – we talk until 2:00 a.m. about health and lots of things. John is working on a Toyota in his garage

August 8 – I fly to Kauai

August 14 – We have a lease signed for the new gallery on Kauai. My health is good but some early vertigo that is stress related

August 15 – My heath has been weak but considering the basic lack of sleep and foreign bed, cannot expect much. Fatigue is prevalent a lot but I feel the problem could be an accumulative effect. I am much more tired than I was a week ago. Work out a lot of the time in the afternoon and evening. Hawaii higher humidity in summer – off my meditation rituals

August 16 – Thom Abott and I check into the Coconut Beach Hotel in Kapaa. I am tired for sure. my bowels have loosened a bit

August 17 – Sleeping well now but still light headed. Heat? Stress? We have been swimming about every day since we arrived on Kauai

August 19 – I call John Thoreson. Thom Abbott and I fly all night with Northwest Airlines. Arrive in Seattle at 5:40 a.m., Wednesday

August 20 – Kim meets me in Seattle

August 24 – No coffee, I have trouble sleeping

August 25 – No coffee. Trouble sleeping again

August 26 – List house for sale for $89,500 – have offer by 5:00 p.m. - $86,000 – we accept

September 7 – We are really deep into packing. Since it is so time consuming, there is nothing else on our agenda

Sept 19 – Go to Seattle. We have our cats immunized for rabies, for the quarantine and move to Kauai. I feel pretty yucky

September 20 – I feel sick

September 21 – I still feel sick – flu-like and MS symptoms. Empty bowels and sensitive stomach

September 22 – I feel better

September 27 – Touch of flu? Bowels emptying

September 28 – Rest all day. Uncomfortable but does not feel like MS. diahhrea

October 11 – Still emptying/packing. My bowels are still erratic

November 11 – We will stay at Judy's house in Port Ludlow for six weeks. Kim and I take the time to build a fence for the cats at Judy's house which is actually for sale

November 27 – We go to my sisters in Vancouver, WA. Watch a movie about Jim Pepper

December 3 – We take another load of crates to Lynden Air Freight in Seattle. My health feels good

December 7 – Meet with John Thoreson. John gives me information about Seriphos

December 12 – I begin taking Seriphos

December 18 – Meet with John Thoreson. John has the beginning of a cold

December 25 – A great time with Mom and Dad, Maryann and Jerrie

December 31 – Cliff Collins takes us to Gary's house with our three cats. We will stay at Gary's overnight

January 1, 1998 – Happy New Year! We fly to Honolulu. The trip went well. We will rent a room from Darlene in Kailua for a month while the cats are in quarantine. We will visit them five days a week. We will become their primary caregivers

January 2 – We go to "Friends" coffee house in Kailua. Home in Hawaii again

January 17 – I call John Thoreson for Seriphos order

January 18 – We go to Ala Moana Center, Honolulu. My health has been great

January 19 – We have dinner at a Chinese restaurant with Darlene

January 20 – I spend the day digesting the dinner we had last night. The meal was tasty but real hard for me to handle

January 31 – We arrive with our three cats on Kauai. The first night on a blow-up mattress with a bubble in the middle was very hard to get any sleep – especially with three cats! Buy a Britta water filter

February 6 – I have to take the day off in Hanapepe while Kim is in the attached house painting the walls. I have caught a cold

February 7 – Carol/Marty Kahn come by to see gallery. They will be returning the art. Marty buys "Demitasse/Gold Ribbon" painting for $450 – a present for Carol

February 9 – Kim comes down with cold

February 13 – Our wedding anniversary – we go to Kalaheo Coffee Company for breakfast. Hanapepe Café for lunch

February 22 – We rest and meditate at Salt Pond Park

February 23 – We go to health food store in Kapaa

March 6 – Grand opening at Kim Starr Gallery. Cliff Collins and Ricky Kelly are playing music. Not a lot of people, but the show went well

March 17 – I have a strong headache all day that runs all night. I had started exercising two days ago again so it may be a self-induced headache

August 31 – Wrote Mom a birthday letter. My health has been somewhat compromised because of stress and Kim being depressed so much. I lay in the back of the gallery I the storage room every chance I get

October 19 – Did not sleep last night. Emptied bowels all night. Could be from too many hours working

October 21 – I am still weak from the last few days of purging

October 23 – We go to Longs Drugs to buy soy milk

October 27 – Kim and I continue to go swimming

October 30 – Even lying down during the day, I am very tired at the end of the day

December 11 – I really overdid things yesterday – I made myself sick. Bad evening just because of fatigue. Pretty dizzy and wobbly. Some diahhrea

December 13 – I quit drinking coffee for a week

January 22, 1999 – I called John Pageler, a man that wrote "New Hope, Real Help for People with MS". John Pageler lives in Florida. John sends out a free news letter every month

January 30 – Overall, my health has been good - I am working too much though. Fatigue for sure – even though I lay down in the storage room a lot

February 13 – Our seventeenth wedding anniversary. We have breakfast in Kalaheo, lunch at Coco's in Wailua

February 14 – I begin working out again with weights. Meditation in morning

March 11 – I take Kim to airport for a mainland trip

March 22 – I feel yucky

November 19 – I am not feeling very well – fatigue **June 17, 2000** – I fly to Seattle. The past seven months have been a continuation of the previous year or so. Kim and I continue to swim a lot, meditate and take care of ourselves. We have become responsible for spaying and neutering stray cats in and around Hanapepe. We now have a route that we take every night to feed stray cats. My health has been even. As I run the art gallery, I find the lack of traffic actually works in one way to an advantage for me. I can lie down, really whenever I need to. The business in Hanapepe is slow but the overhead is also not very high. We cannot afford an employee, so often times I find myself sitting in our kitchen and peering through the doors into the gallery if I open the gallery door. If someone comes in, I go out and greet them. Not much stress on me. If I am in the gallery and Kim is painting in her studio, I can also lay down in a bed I have in the storage room. I have also added a juicer, refrigerator, etc. so I can keep on top of my health. I have a ready stock of kipper snacks, soy milk and soy protein

July 1 – I go to Olympia and visit Danny Spearman. Danny is barely walking. I spend an hour with Danny then head for Fall City

July 3 – John Thoreson ends up in Overlake Hospital in intensive care. I do not hear from him

July 4 – Gary and I leave for airport. I talk with Laura Lee about John. John is okay! Yippee! I fly back to Kauai

July 21 – I receive vitamins/herbs from John Thoreson

July 24 – I buy ten cans of Nature's Plus "Energy" protein. I drink this soy drink with soy milk every morning as well as during the day when I need a boost at the gallery during the day

Sept 12 – I lift weights and do eight Sun Salutes

January 25, 2001 – I have a dizzy day

January 26 – My health is still very slow. I lay down most of the day

February 27 – We leave for Seattle – arrive at 9:30 p.m. There is a riot in Pioneer Square during the Mardi Gras celebration

February 28 – Kim and I have coffee in Carnation, Washington with Gary Daubert. An earthquake runs us out of the building

April 28 – I feel sick in the morning – viral in feeling. Spend the day in bed

April 29 – I feel sketchy but a little better. Take Chinese herbs "Pei Pa Li" and lots of vitamin C

May 5 – Fighting flu virus – 102.5 temperature

May 6 – I stay in bed – 101 degree temperature

May 7 – I stay in bed

May 8 – I stay in bed

May 13 – I have swollen lymph gland in my left groin

May 16 – I go to see Dr. Spear about the lump in my groin. Suggests biopsy in the next two weeks if it does not disappear. I call John Thoreson because I am concerned. John settles me with some good information – I begin to use hydrotherapy. Using hot compresses for three minutes, then cold compresses for two minutes

May 17 – I do more research. Sleep pretty well until 4:00 a.m. Kim and I go to the beach. I walk a lot on the beach and swim – hoping the lump disappears. I constantly check the swelling of my lymph gland. It appears to be shrinking, but I do make an appointment to see Dr. Yarema on Tuesday

May 18 – I take most of the day off – my groin does concern me. I have been doing everything in Linda Page's book "Health Healing" plus John Thoreson's input. By 5:00 p.m. the gland does appear to be shrinking. I really do not have an appetite. I force the issue by eating kipper snack and steamed broccoli. I order Sunrider herbs from Sunrider. My temperature is back to normal. I take most of the day off. I check my lymph gland a lot. I drink lots of filtered water as usual. I am fatigued. I am drinking lemon water to jump start my endocrine system for cleansing

May 22 – Doctors appt with Dr. Yarema. Dr Yarema gives me a homeopathic medicine for "lymph clear". I also start the basic quinary from Sunrider

May 24 – I have night sweats. I turn my bed sheets, wet with sweat. I feel fine but paranoid about the gland. It seems to be puffed up again. Maybe the pain has dissipated a little. Doing my inverted leg exercise on the wall may help the swelling go down

May 26 – I am taking the homeopathic drops. Also, doing a aqua-therapy - hot and cold water alternating

May 27 – I have the night sweats – turn my sheets wet. I have a carrot, beet and ginger drink. I write down ten positive affirmations for the healing of my lymph gland

May 28 – Some tightness and dull pain in gland. Pointed in pain in lymph. Less blue, but red at gland site. Pain keeps me from ignoring it

June 1 – I take the first pill of Doxycycline at 7:00 p.m. Thursday evening. At 9:00 a.m. I take a second Doxycycline. 8:00 p.m. the lymph node is red, swollen and small shots of pain emanating from the gland

June 6 – I go to see Dr. Yarema. The lymph gland is pimpling. Dr Yarema says it will drain soon

June 7 – Less pain from lymph node

June 12 – Kim's birthday. Swelling way down in lymph gland

June 15 – Gland is small but still evident with redness

June 23 – I have been lifting weights for a week now

June 26 – I go to see Dr. Yarema

July 1 – I fly to Seattle

July 9 – I meet John Thoreson at U.S. Biotech – they draw my blood for a screening

July 15 – I fly back to Kauai

July 21 – I quit taking Doxycycline. My groin is still red on the surface, but no swelling or pain for a month

July 27 – Kim has her first colonic

September 11 – The New York twin towers are hit by terrorists

September 28 – More people for Art Night than expected after the bombing of the Twin Towers. We go for a swim

October 5 – I take most of the day off. Not feeling very well. Headache and stiff

October 6 – We go to the beach

October 7 – Work on Social Security five year evaluation

November 29 – We have our teeth cleaned in Hanalei

November 30 – We fly to Honolulu for a signing at the Art Board store at Ala Moana shopping center

December 13 – I am sick with a sore throat

December 14 – I have a bad cold

December 20 – I am in Cold recovery and feel weak and sketchy

December 21 – Fly to Honolulu

December 22 – Neurological exam – Dr Casin

December 25 – Christmas. Kim bakes two vegetable pot pies

January 11, 2002 Stretch, lift weights and meditate

January 27 – Realtors come in and tour building

February 13 – Our 20th wedding anniversary. Plantation Gardens for dinner

February 15 – Go to the beach for a swim

March 16 - Drank coffee/two Lipton teas during the day. I deal with shortness of breath.

March 17 – Spend day in bed with shortness of breath, anxiety and fatigue.

March 18 - I take it easy.

March 20 – Kim has baby tooth pulled.

March 25 – Kim still has pain in gum.

March 30 – I feel yucky.

March 21 – I feel wasted. No coffee

April 1 – I begin taking Sunrider again. Make first car payment on new 2001 Ford Focus.

April 3 – I am feeling better. Sunrider. No coffee

April 4 – My health is still guarded.

April 5 – I have been working out consistently for two weeks. Still fleeting shortness of breath. Some depression. No coffee.

April 6 – My health is okay. No coffee. Still shortness of breath.

April 10 – Dad's birthday. We are moving to Maui. There is an accepted offer on this Hanapepe property we just rent.

April 21 – We fly to Maui.

June 12 – Kim's forty-sixth birthday. Kim hosts party with Judi, Karen, Kim and I. Kim makes two cakes. One lemon and one chocolate. Plus salads and manna bread. I give Kim the "Space boy" trash can for a present.

June 18 – I did not sleep very well but have been sleeping better the last few nights.

October 3 – I feel rough. Empty bowels.

October 8 – We receive termination of lease. Have forty-five days to move. We have to be out by November 23. Lots of stress. No sleep.

October 8 – We pack our house and our gallery.

October 24 – We fly to Maui to look for a place to live.

October 27 – Return from rental search on Maui.

November 10 – Fatigue

November 12 – Packing almost complete. Stress!!

January 1, 2003 – We are living in Kula, Maui.

January 10 – Kim and I take laundry to Pukalani. We hand in our offer to Lease at Ma'alaea Shops. We are waiting for FedEx to deliver 16" stainless steel balls.

February 9 – We put up a 10x20 tent in front yard for room to paint beach ball sculpture.

February 11 – John Papazian shows the property we are renting.

February 13 – Our 21st wedding anniversary. We buy stainless steel table at Costco.

February 15 – Our tent blows down in front yard.

April 23 – Kim and I have been struggling with our present situation. Both living and working. Very difficult to produce while living in the concrete bunker with 6 cats and boxes. The gallery proposal at Ma'alaea Harbor still has no resolve.

April 24 – The landlord calls. People are touring the property here again today. The property may be sold. We would have until August 1 to move.

April 26 – Go to Wailea Beach to photograph Sculpture.

May 3 – Left leg problem still bothersome. I injured my leg exercising too hard.

May 5 – Chiropractor appt. in Makawao

May 6 – My sciatic nerve on left side is real tender.

May 7 – I have been icing the left leg several times a day. My sciatic nerve feels better.

June 1 – The rental in Makawao falls through at the last minute. We have eleven days to move. We decide to move to the mainland to buy a house and to be closer to Mom and Dad. So much work and anxiety. Kim is painting on 50x60 oil (Aqua/White Beach ball)

June 2 - Kim is painting. I have made thirty phone calls to arrange the move

June 4 – We have no hot water in Kula. Container is sitting at the front door. We are packing big time

June 5 – We buy cat containers. We take baths by pouring hot water over our heads from the stove

June 8 – We finish packing container, take ramp apart

June 9 – Go to Matson Navigation, pay for container. Meet Audie Lam at Starbucks

June 10 – Kim and I have coffee in Makawao. Beautiful day in Makawao. Audie comes by in evening to pick up air conditioner

June 11 – Kim and I sleep on empty floor in Kula – drop cloth and futon. What a night. We take two boxes to the mail with bedding. We then leave for Matson to drop off car. Arrive at 10:00a.m. with three cat containers full of 6 cats. Catch cab to airport. At check in, the Hawaiian Airlines ticket clerk asks for our health certificates. What?! We had no idea about this. Would not let us on the flight without the certificates. From there they insist on certificates. I have to call a mobile vet to come to the Kahului airport to check out our cats. When he arrives and we pay him $290 with a Visa, he looks at the six cats through the cages and writes up the certificates. Hawaiian Air could not even provide a room for the Vet to do a proper exam. So he just visualized the cat's curbside. The next hurdle was Hawaiian Airlines would not let two cats in a container Maximum 1 cat per container. They literally went back on their rules of which I had been on the phone with them three different times. I had reservations for these cats just the way they were. Two in each container. The supervisor decided to let us go if we would go get three more containers and load the cats each in a container. Off we go. We are cleared to go. We take off in a new Boeing 767. A very smooth flight. Kim and I have Lion coffee on the plane at 4:00 p.m. Wow, how delicious. We now know we will land in Seattle. We arrived at 2:00 a.m. Nobody around. We rent a Chevy Blazer. We miss the Bainbridge Island ferry so have to drive over the Narrows Bridge. What a trip. We arrive at our home for the next two months in Port Angeles at 4:00 a.m.

June 25 – Sleeping well these days. Beautiful weather in the Northwest. I take Dad for an eye doctor appointment in Olympia.

June 27 – We meet a truck driver at our storage in Port Townsend. We spend the next 7 hours with a friend unloading the 24ft. container.

June 28 – We spend 3.5 more hours to finish unloading the 24 ft. container into our third storage unit

June 29 – I rest and sleep

June 30 – I call dispatcher to pick up empty container

July 1 – I take Mom to Tacoma for sewing machine repair

July 5 – I am catching a virus

July 6 – I am sick with a high fever – rough day

July 8 – I have a bad cold

July 10 – The cold has changed course somewhat to chest. I am coughing a lot

July 11 – I awaken at 5:00 a.m. with uncontrollable cough

July 13 – Kim has cold! My cold is way into my chest but hopefully fading

July 14 – We sign Earnest money for our house in Snoqualmie

July 15 – Rest. Our colds are very present

July 22 – Meet building inspector at house in Snoqualmie

July 23 – We recover from exhausting day. 200 mile drive, stress, and just too much. We are in tears. 7:00 p.m. we recover laying around in the yard with the cats. A branch falls in the yard in the evening ad collapses part of our cat pen

July 24 – I wake at 4:00 a.m. but go back to sleep

August 1 – I drive to Gary Dauberts. We will leave for Mom and Dad's at Hood Canal in the morning. We will take a load of boxes to Vancouver, WA where they are moving

August 8 – Kim and I go to the Port Angeles Starbucks. A second cup of coffee – mistake. We are meditating again regularly

August 14 – We have been on the mainland 60 days now. Our house purchase is going fine, appraisal fine

August 18 – Gary and I leave for Mom and Dad's house. We pick up wood stove and range, etc.

August 20 – We go to Port Townsend storage

August 22 – We leave for Bellevue and sign our closing papers on our house in Snoqualmie

August 23 – Rest and clean trailer in Port Angeles. Pack and ready to move out completely in the morning

August 24 – We move to Snoqualmie – all six cats on board. Full car even the roof rack!! Arrive in Snoqualmie at 1:30 p.m. We leave the cats in bedroom while we go to the food co-op. We will all sleep in the room until we clean the new house somewhat

August 25 – Gorgeous weather. We leave for North Bend Starbucks to meet Gary

August 29 – We start working on the front yard fence in our new home in Snoqualmie

August 31 – Gary brings his chainsaw over. We cut the credenza in the kitchen in thirds and haul it away

September 4 – We leave in the early morning for Hood canal to help Mom and Dad move. This is their last day at the Canal – a very sad say. The end of an era. Also Mom's 84th birthday. Dad told me he was really going to miss the Canal – very sad

September 5 – A beautiful 90 degree day. Gary hooks a chain to the stump in the backyard and pulls it out with his truck

September 9 – I order new glasses. My frames have been broken for over a week. Now it will be a couple of weeks without glasses

September 17 – My sciatic nerve in my left leg is bothersome. We rented a U-haul truck and head for Port Townsend storage. My back is also tweaked from moving

September 22 – Kim and I start drinking Essiac tea in the evenings again. Bill Rooney made the tea for us! We had purchased the Essiac at the food co-op in Port Townsend. 5:30 p.m. meditation

October 5 – My left sciatic nerve is still painful – I wake up with pain

October 6 – I still have left leg pain

October 7 – I have a cold. Not bad yet – runny nose type. Pain in my leg is lighter

October 8 – I have a chiropractic appointment in North Bend

October 12 – Kim has the cold that was passed to me from Gary

October 31 – Crystal clear and 20 degrees outside

December 2 – We take Piedmont to vet eye specialist for scratched eye

December 13 – I move tree rounds from Steve's downed tree across the street and strain my left shoulder

December 14 – Sadaam Hussein is captured

December 23 – We design/paint beach ball ornaments to give away as Christmas presents

December 24 – We leave for Mom and Dad's in Vancouver, Washington to spend Christmas with them

December 31 – New Years eve

January 1, 2004 – Snowing in Snoqualmie – gorgeous! My left shoulder is not getting any better

January 2 – Beautiful, snowy weather. The sun came out a little

January 3 – Kim is prepping canvases

January 4 – Cold and windy

January 5 – 12 degrees outside, windy!

January 6 – Cold, snow – Kim and I go for a walk – I fall on the icy road

January 7 – Cold and wind. Kim and I try to walk to the store – too slippery!

January 8 – Snow is melting. I shovel some snow

January 10 – Kim is on day two of a 30x40 oil painting

January 11 – Beautiful weather and 40 degrees!

January 13 – Kim goes skating for the first time since moving to Snoqualmie

January 21 – We pick up cousin, Jim Macfarland in Seattle and drive south to meet with Mom and Dad in Centralia area

January 30 – My left arm is still pretty difficult to straighten over my head. An injury incurred by lifting the log rounds from across the street

February 6 – I begin writing my book about my life with MS

February 7 – I have swollen glands and scratchy throat

February 9 – Beautiful day – 44 degrees. I have cold. The sun shows up

February 10 – I am a little better but my skin hurts

February 11 – 50 degrees outside – blue sky. My cold is better

February 12 – Kim has a cold. Beautiful day outside – beautiful flowers

February 13 (Friday) – Our 22nd wedding anniversary. I take MSM in evening because of my stiff left arm

February 15 -0 Kim has cold. We meet with *John Thoreson*. He gives us a jar of Amla for our immune system. Loans us a couple of books

February 16 – We meet with JoAnne Etheridge in Bellevue for lunch at the Cheesecake Factory. I order fish tacos

February 20 – My arm still bothers me when moved a certain way

February 22 – Kim and I walk to river – beautiful and 60 degrees

February 23 – My left arm still aches. I have been taking MSM for over a week. I cannot raise my arm much higher than my lower chest. Actually, the arm is really starting to ache a lot. I cannot sleep on this side anymore

February 24 – We go to Seattle. Kim skates. Tired at end of day

February 25 – We take Elliot to eye doctor in Bellevue. My arm is bothersome – hard to sleep

February 28 – Kim works on paint booth in shop

February 29 – Kim works in paint booth. Arm might be a little less painful but still cannot lift higher than middle shoulder

March 1 – Overcast but beautiful

March 4 – Kahn Galleries sells "Model with Purse" oil painting. John Thoreson calls and is in Port Townsend and visiting *Douwe Rienstra*. Tells Douwe about book.

March 5 – I have chiropractic appt. *Dr. Piffner* refers me to a physical therapist

March 6 – Kim paints 22" beach ball sculpture

March 9 – Kim goes ice skating. We feed John's cat, Odin on the way home

March 10 – My first physical therapy appt

March 11 – Tough night sleep because of arm. My sister Jerrie's birthday

March 19 – Set up Seattle trade show at Convention center

March 28 – We go to Port Townsend and empty 10x10 storage unit

March 30 – Kim goes skating. We stop at Western Neon

March 31 – We take sculpture to Western Neon. Also, physical therapy. Pain

April 2 – Exercises at home increased to 2 minute holds on each stretch

April 7 – Kim photographs Beach Ball sculpture. I am at physical therapy. Add an exercise. I mow lawn. I slept okay. Sleep has been difficult for a couple of months. Not being able to sleep or turn on left shoulder

April 8 – I add a stick to my arm exercises - to push left hand from right side

April 9 – Kim is baking a four tier cake for Dad's 87th birthday

April 14 – I have gastric problem. I wonder if this is from our meal in Centralia? A fish sandwich. I feel real rough in the stomach

April 16 – I feel better in the lower gut

April 18 – I have the diarrhea again. I shall quit fish oil capsules for a few days

April 19 – My 54th birthday. Kim makes s a four tier cake. We go to Krispy Kreme – we buy mug and shirt – no donuts

April 24 – We go to Seattle to see skating competition. Come home and mow lawn. We go for a walk in evening as usual

May 2 – (Sunday) My shoulder is still frozen, but I am working on it more and more since the pain has subsided

May 3 – 80 degrees outside. I work on front yard grass strip

May 15 – Kim has first group ice-skating lesson

May 17 – Kim has a cold

May 19 – Mom and Dad's 59th wedding anniversary. We have to cancel our trip to Vancouver because of Kim's virus

May 24 – I am still doing left arm exercises. Also icing the shoulder. Much less pain but still movement inhibited

May 26 – I walk to Snoqualmie Falls and back – two mile round trip

May 28 – Kim is painting in Candy's room. I am working on book. Rain. Health fine

May 29 – We pick up John Thoreson at 7:00 a.m. and head for Seattle

May 30 – I walk to Snoqualmie Falls in fifty minutes. Kim is painting. I am working on book

May 31 – Memorial Day. We have two tomatoes on our plants

June 1 – Shoulder exercises daily

June 2 – I walk to Falls and back home – 57 minutes

June 3 – Shoulder is stressed. Deliver gravel to backyard for posts

June 4 – Kim is painting. John Thoreson climbs Mt. Si

June 5 – Pick up John at 7:00 a.m. – go to Seattle. Morning at Elliot Bay Book Store. For six days I have been able to sleep on my stomach. I feel the shoulder but okay to sleep. I am also able to put fingers in my left back pocket like the physical therapist suggested

June 6 – I walk to Snoqualmie Falls for the fourth time. I am also reading more books on MS. Heavy rain for an hour in the afternoon

June 7 – I help Gary cut firewood in the rain

June 12 – Kim's birthday! Go ice skating. Lunch at Sunlight restaurant

June 14 – I walk to Falls in morning for fifth day in a row

June 16 – Beautiful weather. Physical therapy, more movement. Right index finger has been twitching off and on for three days

June 18 – 90 degrees yesterday. Another beautiful day. Index finger has spasm for five days

June 20 – 100 degrees in shade

June 24 – Put six more posts in concrete in backyard

June 26 – Kim has skating class. My shoulder is getting better slowly. Pain has overall diminished again. I can sleep on left shoulder and have for two weeks now. So, I have been enjoying better sleep!

June 28 – Pick cherries for the third time

July 4 – Independence Day!

July 5 – I walk to Falls

July 12 – Stringing fencing

July 15 – I have flu-like symptoms in afternoon

July 16 – I spend day mostly in bed with food poisoning (?) Kim and I had spent two days with Mom and Dad in Vancouver, Wash. I have diahhrea and uncomfortable symptoms

July 17 – Kim skates. I rest all morning I car. Still feeling sick. Now weak

July 18 – I feel better for sure. The weather has been wonderful

July 21 – Toothache

July 22 – Toothache

July 23 – 102 degrees in the sun at 5:00 p.m.

July 25 – Cooler. Work on fence. I still have toothache. I don't know if top right tooth or bottom right

July 26 – Kim and I meet person in Seattle. I have quite an intense toothache. I take an Ibuprofen and a Pei Pa Li. Have found some relief but still a problem of significant pain

July 27 – I have dentist appt. at 2:00 p.m. John Thoreson is on his way to Portland. Dentist sends me to a specialist. Fortunately able to see Dr. Pratten in

Issaquah this afternoon. Runs tests to figure out which tooth. Nothing definitive

July 28 – I am sure of which tooth is the problem now – top right!

July 29 – I have two hour appt. for a root canal. Amazing dentist – really no pain at6 all. Beautiful weather. Kim finishes pastel of JoAnne's cat Toby

July 30 – No tooth pain

July 31 – Neither Kim nor I sleep very well. Full moon (?) Put up last six boards of fence in backyard

August 1 – JoAnne and Chuck's wedding party in Port Townsend. Fill car with storage stuff

August 2 – Kim gets ready for her trip to Kauai

August 3 – I take Kim to airport

August 4 – Working on Florida representation

August 6 – Go to Port Townsend with John Thoreson. Fill car with storage stuff

August 8 – Kim and Catharine visit Hanapepe Hill cats. I work outside all day. 80 degrees today – perfect

August 11 – I have physical therapy appt. Really nothing more he can do for me until I have more time to improve

August 12 – Kim arrives home at 9:45 p.m. – yippee! We stay up until 2:30 a.m.

August 18 – I have crown measurement dental appt. Kim is working in studio. 80 degrees outside

August 19 – Kim is in studio in morning. I work on book. String fence in backyard in afternoon. 80 degrees outside

August 22 – Meet Gary's new girlfriend. Rain last night. Spend afternoon with John Thoreson on book

August 23 – Rain hard. Have chimney repair estimate

August 24 – We go to Seattle for Kim's weekly ice skating practice

August 25 – I life weights. No movement of left arm yet since injury. Have been lifting off and on for several months. My left arm is lengthing in stretch

August 27 – I have dentist appt. for two hours for a crown prep. Kim is painting. Lots of rain over the last two days but still 70 degrees

August 28 – We go to National Dahlia show to see our neighbor's entry, etc. Max has been growing dahlias for twenty years. This is a big show for him. At the Hilton, near the airport

August 30 – Chimney repair is finished. Kim varnishes paintings. We send two original pastels of Carole and Marty's dog and cat to Kahn Galleries

August 31 – Beautiful 80 degree weather. Kim skates in Seattle

September 1 – Kim is painting.

September 2 – Lift weights in morning and stretch as usual. I go to Gary's and pick Japanese pears. They are wonderful

September 3 – Overcast day with 60's weather. Headed to John Thoreson's house to work on book.

The last entry into this timeline marks a significant date. Fourteen years ago today on September 3, 1990 I experienced an exacerbation that really began my life with Multiple Sclerosis. I continue writing in a journal.

Every day is a gift.

Chapter

15

Reference Materials

These books happen to be on the shelf next to this computer. Some are my favorites. I rely on them to this day. Others I read and shelved. When I started to amass websites via these books, the task became overwhelming – much like the internet itself.

1. *CREATING HEALTH* by Dr. Deepak Chopra c.1987 Houghton Mifflin Company www.chopra.com

2. *QUANTUM HEALING* by Dr. Deepak Chopra c.1989 Bantam Books www.chopra.com

3. *PERFECT HEALTH* by Dr. Deepak Chopra c.1991 Harmony Books, a division of Crow Publishers, Inc. www.chopra.com

4. *THE I CHING or BOOK OF CHANGES; a guide to life's turning points* by Brian Browne Walker c.1992 Brian Browne Walker, St. Martin's Press

5. *HEALING MULTIPLE SCLEROSIS* by Anne Boroch c.2007 Quintessential Healing, Inc. Publishing www.annboroch.com

6. *THE MULTIPLE SCLEROSIS DIET BOOK* by Dr. Roy Laver Swank c.1997, 1987 Published by Doubleday www.swankmsdiet.com

7. *NEW HOPE REAL HELP FOR PEOPLE WITH MS* by John Pageler, out of print

8. *HANDBOOK OF MULTIPLE SCLEROSIS* by Khurram Bashir, M.D. and John N. Whitaker, M.D. c.2002 Lippinccott Williams and Wilkins

9. *MULTIPLE SCLEROSIS- THE QUESTIONS YOU HAVE, THE ASNWERS YOU NEED* by Rosalind C. Kalb, PhD c.2000 Demos Medical Publishing, Inc.

10. *MULTIPLE SCLEROSIS – THE FACTS YOU NEED* by Dr. Paul O'Connor MD c.1999 Firefly books

11. *MULTIPLE SCLEROSIS a Guide for Patients and Their Families* edited by: Labe C. Scheinberg, M.D. c.1983 Raven Press Books

12. *MULTIPLE SCLERISIS* by Louis J. Rosner M.D. and Shelley Ross c.1987 Fireside, a registered trademark of Simon and Schuster

13. *LIVING BEYOND MULTIPLE SCLEROSIS;A WOMAN'S GUIDE* by Judith Lynn Nichols c.2000 Judith Lynn Nichols Hunter House Publishers www.hunterhouse.com

14. *MONEY DRIVEN MEDICINE* by Maggie Mahar c. 2006 Maggie Mahar HarpperCollins books

15. *THE POWER OF POSITIVE THINKING* by Norman Vincent Peale

16. *THE WELLNESS REVOLUTION* by Paul Zane Pilzer c. 2002 John Wiley/Sons Inc. Hoboken N.J.

17. *DENTISTRY WITHOUT MERCURY* by Sam Ziff and Michael F. Ziff D.D.S. c. 1985 by Bio Probe, Inc. www.bioprobe.com

18. *ANTIOXIDANTS AGAINST CANCER* by Ralph W. Moss PhD. C.2000 Equinox Press www.cancerdecisions.com

19. *THE WHEATGRASS BOOK* by Ann Wigmore c. 1985 Ann Wigmore and Hippocrates Health Institute, Inc. Avery Publishing; a member of Penguin Putnam Inc. www.annwigmore.com

20. *SUPER SUPPLEMENTS* by Michael E. Rosenbaum, M.D. and Dominick Bosco c.1987 Penguin Group

21. *MULTIPLE SCLEROSIS Q&A REASSURING ANSWERS TO FREQUENTLY ASKED QUESTIONS* by Beth Ann Hill c. 2003 Avery; a member of Penguin Group

22. *REVERSING MULTIPLE SCLEROSIS* by Celeste Pepe, D.D., N. D. and Lisa Hammond c. 2001 Hampton Roads Publishing Co. Inc

Note: I have read countless other books and articles. I continue to learn about life, spirituality in healing and Multiple Sclerosis.

Chapter

In Closing. . . . .

I am no different than anyone else. I endeavor to live a happy, productive life. Writing this book has given me the opportunity to offer you the benefit of my experience.

For those of you who have MS, please take these words as encouragement to learn all you can about MS. Do not hand your health over to someone you feel may know more than you about this disease.

Be a participant in your healing. You and your loved ones will be happy you did.

www.ingramcontent.com/pod-product-compliance
Lightning Source LLC
Chambersburg PA
CBHW060356290526
45791CB00002B/528